the functions
of the
orgasms

Michel Odent is best known as the obstetrician who introduced the concepts of birthing pools and home-like birthing rooms. He has published 12 books in 21 languages and recently completed a trilogy of books, *The Scientification of Love*, *The Farmer and the Obstetrician*, and *The Caesarian*. His other books include *Birth Reborn* and *Birth and Breastfeeding*.

the functions of the orgasms

of the
orgasms

THE HIGHWAYS TO
TRANSCENDENCE

MICHEL ODENT

PINTER & MARTIN

The Functions of the Orgasms
The Highways to Transcendence

First published in Great Britain by Pinter & Martin Ltd 2009

ISBN 978-1-905177-18-9

British Library Cataloguing-in-Publication Data
A catalogue record for this book is available from the British Library

Set in Garamond

Printed and bound in Great Britain by
Athenaeum Press Ltd, Gateshead, Tyne & Wear

This book has been printed on paper that is sourced and
harvested from sustainable forests and is FSC accredited

Pinter & Martin Ltd
6 Effra Parade
London SW2 1PS

www.pinterandmartin.com

CONTENTS

1

THE TOP OF THE LADDERS

Every episode of human sexual life can reach a climax. It helps to recall that the Greek word 'climax' originally means 'ladder'. Every ladder has a culminant point. This book is about the top of the ladders.

We'll focus on three particular situations, looking first at the 'fetus ejection reflex', before considering male and female orgasms in genital sexuality, and also the milk ejection reflex. Our objective is to go beyond the easy-to-explain roles of these varieties of climax, during which either the sperm is transported towards the egg at the time of conception, or the baby is pushed through the maternal genital path during the birth process, or the milk is ejected during lactation. We'll look at these climaxes as intense responses at all levels of the nervous-endocrine system, as changes of conscious levels, as possible ways to escape from daily space and time reality and to reach transcendent emotional states.

We shall not hesitate to use the word 'orgasm'. This is a way to wink at the pioneering work of Wilhelm Reich, who was audacious enough to publish *The Function of the Orgasm* in the scientific context of the 1940s.[1] At that time such a word was still taboo, although Aphra Behn – the first Englishwoman credited with earning her livelihood by authorship – introduced it in English language as early as 1684: in *The Disappointment* she describes the woman's emotional state after a failure to achieve 'orgasm'. Our objective is to a certain extent to rewrite *The Function of the Orgasm* in a new scientific context. This will lead us to enlarge the topic. Wilhelm Reich focused on genital sexuality although he was aware of the work of Helen Deutsch – the first woman doctor graduated at the University of Vienna and member of the Vienna Psycho-Analytic society. Helen Deutsch, who had the experience of giving birth and breastfeeding, considered sexual intercourse and giving birth as two phases of one process divided only by a time interval: 'Just as the first act contains an element of the second, so the second is impregnated with pleasure mechanisms of the first. I even believe that the act of birth represents the acme of sexual pleasure...' Furthermore, according to her, breastfeeding is 'an act of sexual enjoyment, at the heart of which the mammary gland plays the part of an erogenous zone.'[2]

We'll also enlarge the topic by occasional allusions to the similarities between orgasmic states and other ecstatic states. Such similarities remained ignored in modern Western cultures until recently, although they were taken for granted in Eastern cultures in the age of female Tantric Masters, and elsewhere in the age of sacred prostitutes.[3] Una Kroll is one of those who have eloquently highlighted the links between a great diversity of ecstatic states. Having been a nun, a medical doctor, a priestess and the mother of four children, she could authoritatively write: 'Moments of ecstasy have recurred like grace notes throughout my life... The ecstasy of sexual union is akin to that of ecstatic prayer...'[4]

Aphra Behn, Helen Deutsch and Una Kroll have at least one thing in common: they are all women. Similarly, after becoming a mother, Niles Newton was the first scientist who anticipated, as early as the 1950s, that oxytocin has behavioral effects.[5] Until that time only the mechanical effects of that hormone had been considered, particularly the effects on uterine contractions making the birth of the baby and of the placenta possible, and the effects on specialized cells of the breast, making the milk ejection reflex possible. Today the role of oxytocin appears as central in all orgasmic and ecstatic states. Today oxytocin appears as the main component of the 'cocktail of love hormones' released during any episode of our sexual life. This observation of the paramount role of women in our understanding of orgasmic states also leads us to recall how Candace Pert demonstrated in 1973 the existence of opiate receptors in the brain: she had paved the way to the discovery of the natural opiates commonly called endorphins.[6] This was an important step in our interpretation of ecstatic states in general. It was also in the 1970s that Regina Lederman published her studies about the inhibitory effects of hormones of the adrenaline family on the birth process.[7]

We must also include among the list of such female trailblazers the name of Kerstin Uvnäs-Moberg, a mother of four children. Her team of researchers at the Karolinska Institute in Stockholm is arguably the most active and productive one in the world where the properties of oxytocin are concerned. What makes this research team unique is that all its members are mothers. Anne Marie Widstrom, Eva Nissen, Anna Berit Ransjo-Arvidson, Ksenia Bystrova, Wibke Jonas, Ingela Wiklund, Marianne Welandria, Anne Sofi Matthiesen, Berit Sjogren, and Maria Pettersson all had the experience of giving birth.

It seems obvious that many women spontaneously perceive the importance of issues that have not traditionally attracted the attention of male dominated scientific circles. It is as if there are female ways to evaluate the comparative importance of different perspectives in exploring human nature. All scientific hypotheses are more or less based on intuitive knowledge and intuitive knowledge is gender related. Until recently the scientific world was highly dominated by men. We are entering a new phase in the history of sciences, with a more symmetrical input from each gender. This new phase is associated with the advent of the 'scientification of love'.[8] Love was traditionally a topic for poets, novelists and philosophers. Today it is studied from multiple scientific perspectives. In such a context it is becoming impossible to refer to love and to raise questions about the development of the capacity to love without keeping in mind the importance of the period surrounding birth. All the disciplines involved in the 'scientification of love' suggest that maternal love is the prototype for all facets of love. The prerequisite for the development of such a vital aspect of the scientific revolution is a more symmetrical gender complementarity and collaboration.

There are several reasons why we'll first look at the fetus ejection reflex. The first reason is that after thousands of years of culturally controlled childbirth very few people – including the natural childbirth advocates – can imagine what it is about. Another reason is that, in the current scientific context, when the fetus ejection reflex is understood, it is easier to look at the other orgasmic/ecstatic states. We must add that this climax probably corresponds to the top of the highest possible ladder human beings may have the opportunity to climb. It is also usually the most highly disturbed and repressed facet of the human orgasmic power. Furthermore we must take into account that our primary objective has been to rewrite *The Function of the Orgasm* in the context of the twenty-first century. This is why we'll choose to start with what Wilhelm Reich could not easily perceive in the early 1940s, that is the similarities between the act of birth and the orgasms of genital sexuality.

Studying the functions of orgasms in the age of the 'scientification of love' inevitably involves referring to recent technical advances, which are making 'love hormones' useless. For example, the cesarean operation has become easier, faster and safer than ever. Furthermore, we now have at our disposal safe and effective pharmacological substitutes for the hormones women are actually programmed to release while giving birth. This is why humanity is in an unprecedented situation. Until recently, even though all cultures dramatically disturb the physiological processes, a woman was obliged to rely on the release of a complex cocktail of love hormones in order to have babies. Today the number of human mothers who rely on their own hormones to birth the baby and the placenta is becoming negligible. At such a turning point in the history of mankind, anybody who is interested in the future of our species should be focused on just one question: 'How long will the human race be able to survive without love?'

2

EXPLORING THE ULTIMATE STEPS OF THE BIRTH LADDER

It happened in a London hospital. A woman was about to give birth to her first baby. A student midwife, an experienced doula and the father were invisible and silent, sharing the sacredness of the moment. At the very time when the ecstatic mother-to-be, who was standing up, started to say 'What a pleasure!', 'It's like making love', 'The baby is coming', and at the precise moment when the perineum started moving, the door suddenly burst open. A female doctor entered the room, shouting: 'I need to make an assessment. You must lie down on the table'. The birthing woman repeated, in an imploring tone: 'Please, please, I beg you, I beg you…' Some time later a drip of synthetic oxytocin was necessary to get the baby out… It is easy to interrupt an orgasm.

Very few health professionals know – or can even imagine – what a birth can be like. From the end of 1953 leading into 1954, I spent six months as an 'externe' (a medical student with minor clinical responsibilities) at the maternity unit of the Hôpital Boucicaut in Paris. My colleagues and I were occasionally given the opportunity to sit in the chief obstetrician's office in the presence of the chief midwife, the most powerful, fearsome, and unnerving person in the unit. During this encounter we were supposed to ask the doctor about particular issues relating to pregnancy and childbirth. I imagine how the doctor would have responded if I'd asked: 'Can giving birth be an ecstatic experience?' or 'Can a birthing place become a sacred place?' The doctor would probably have sent me to the local psychiatrist.

The emergence of new perspectives

Today, more and more articles, conferences, documentaries, and books are openly referring to the idea of ecstatic or orgasmic birth and to the sacredness of childbirth. In 1982 a BBC television crew paid a visit to the French hospital where I was practicing. During the visit a young woman gave birth to her first baby, which happened to be breech. An hour or two after the event the well-known BBC presenter Esther Rantzen asked the mother how she'd felt when the baby had arrived. The mother opened her big, expressive eyes and simply replied: 'It was like an orgasm!' Another woman once told me: 'When I looked at my baby's eyes for the first time, just after the birth, I saw the whole universe in her eyes.' Sarah Buckley – an Australian medical doctor who gave birth to her four children at home – has combined such anecdotes with her personal experience so as to popularize the concept of 'ecstatic birth'.[1]

Considering this sudden emergence of a new perspective on childbirth, we must first note that all known societies have dramatically disturbed the physiological processes relating to childbirth for thousands of years. Cultures interfere mostly by passing on from generation to generation beliefs and rituals. The turning point of the 1970s was immensely significant, not least because of its timing.

It is necessary first of all to use the language and perspective of modern physiologists in order to offer plausible and valuable interpretations. The physiological is a reference point that is independent of culture, unlike the concept of normality. It is impossible to explore deviations from physiological reference points in different cultures without remembering the ideal suggested by modern scientific perspectives. Recent spectacular advances in physiology provide us with the keys to rediscovering the ultimate steps of the birth ladder after thousands of years of culturally controlled childbirth.

The fetus ejection reflex

Climbing the ultimate steps of the birth ladder is the same as giving birth by means of a 'fetus ejection reflex'. This term was coined by Niles Newton in the 1960s when she was studying the environmental factors that can disturb the birth process in mice.[2] Twenty years later, with her support[3] I suggested that we save this concept from oblivion; I was convinced it could be a key to triggering a radically new understanding of the process of human parturition.[4]

The basic difference between humans and mice is that we have developed a huge and powerful new brain (called 'the neocortex'), which covers the archaic structures that we share with all other mammals. When our neocortex is at rest we have more physiological similarities with mice.

An authentic fetus ejection reflex takes place when a human baby is born after a short series of irresistible contractions, which leave no room for voluntary movements. In such circumstances it is obvious that the neocortex (the part of the brain related to intellectual activities) is at rest and no longer in control of the archaic brain structures in charge of vital functions such as giving birth. Civilized women can behave in a way which would usually be unacceptable: they may shout, swear, or be rude, for example. They seem to cut themselves off from our world, and may even forget what they have been taught or what their previous plans were. During a fetus ejection reflex, women can find themselves in the most unexpected, bizarre, often mammalian, quadrupedal postures. They seem to be 'on another planet'. At the very time of the birth and during the minutes following birth, at the beginning of the interaction with the newborn baby, these mothers seem to be in an ecstatic state.

Interpreting the fetus ejection reflex leads us to understand the reduction of the activity of the new big brain as the solution Nature found to overcome the specifically human handicap during the period surrounding birth: one of the reasons why human birth is difficult, compared with birth of other mammals, is precisely the huge development in our species of the neocortex. Such development of the 'brain of the intellect' is a handicap in several contexts because it is the source of inhibitions during the birth process and also during any other kind of sexual experience.

Climbing towards the ultimate steps

There are several reasons why the human fetus ejection reflex has been ignored until recently. The main reason is that the basic needs of laboring women climbing towards the ultimate steps of the birth ladder are almost never met. Their needs are not met because they are not understood. However, we are in a position today to explain what these needs are: a laboring woman needs to feel protected against any stimulation of her neocortex.[5] Since language is a specifically human stimulant of the 'big brain', this leads us to rediscover the importance of silence. When a woman is in labor language should be used only when it is absolutely necessary and with extreme caution. It will take a long time to rediscover the importance of silence and to accept that the dominant quality of a midwife should be her capacity to keep her mouth shut.

Light is also a well-known stimulant of the neocortex. There is a well known 'darkness hormone' called melatonin. Our pineal gland releases this hormone at night to reduce the activity of our neocortex and fall asleep. These are important considerations in the age of electricity. We might add that sight is the most intellectual of our senses. It is noticeable that spontaneously, when women are not influenced by what they read or what they have been taught, they often find postures that tend to eliminate all visual stimulation, e.g. on all fours, as if praying.

Feeling observed, and therefore judged, is a situation that tends to activate the neocortex. This is what we can conclude from common sense and scientific studies. It is also difficult for many people to understand that privacy, in other words not feeling observed, is a basic need. In books and conferences about 'natural childbirth', the most 'unnatural' situations for giving birth are usually portrayed: two or three people (plus a camera!) are positioned in front of the mother-to-be. It is now commonplace to claim that when one observes a phenomenon one transforms it. This is particularly true in the case of basic vital functions such as parturition.

The perception of a possible danger is another typical situation that implies attention and alertness, therefore stimulation of the neocortex. In other words the laboring woman needs to feel secure.

Understanding that laboring women need to feel secure, without feeling observed and judged, leads us to the root of midwifery. It seems that women have always had a tendency to give birth close to their mother, or occasionally close to an experienced mother who could fulfill the role of a mother figure: the midwife was originally a mother figure and, in an ideal world, our mother is the prototype of the person with whom one can feel secure without feeling observed, or judged. In most societies, though, the role of the midwife has been gradually altered. Most languages condition women to accept that they do not have the power to give birth by themselves: they must 'be delivered' by somebody. As a result the midwife has gradually become a figure who is more often that not an authoritarian and dominating guide, an observer, and an agent of the cultural milieu. She has also played a key role in the transmission of perinatal beliefs and rituals.

A crucial moment

It is precisely when birth seems to be imminent that birth attendants have a tendency to become even more intrusive and this is another reason why the human fetus ejection reflex has been ignored until recently. People who can understand the concept of the fetus ejection reflex know that, in optimal physiological conditions, there is an obvious explosive release of high levels of 'catecholamines' (hormones of the adrenaline family) during the very last contractions. A woman who has previously been rather passive suddenly appears to be full of energy; she tends to move into an upright position and often displays a need to grasp something or somebody. For example, if the woman was previously on her hands and knees, her chest tends to become vertical. Other women stand up to give birth, more often than not leaning on the edge of a piece of furniture. A fetus ejection reflex is usually associated with a bending forward posture.

Another symptom of the release of hormones in the adrenaline family is the sudden expression of a fear, with a frequent reference to death. The woman may say: 'Am I going to die?' 'Kill me!' or 'Let me die...'[6] Instead of keeping a low profile, the well-intentioned birth attendants usually interfere, at least with reassuring rational words. These rational words can interrupt the progress towards the fetus ejection reflex. This reflex does not occur if there is a birth attendant who behaves like a 'coach', or an observer, or a helper, or a guide, or a 'support person'.[7] It is exceptionally rare if the baby's father participates in the birth. The fetus ejection reflex can also be inhibited by vaginal examinations, eye-to-eye contact or by the imposition of a change of environment, as would happen when a woman is transferred to a delivery room. It is inhibited when the intellect of the laboring woman is stimulated by any sort of rational language, for example if the birth attendant says: 'Now you are at complete dilation. It's time to push.' In other words, any interference tends to bring the laboring woman 'back down to Earth' and tends to transform the fetus ejection reflex into a second stage of labor which involves voluntary movements.[8] Those who understand the fetus ejection reflex realize how useless it is to exchange views with others on issues such as breech birth,[9] posterior position of the baby's head,[10] shoulder dystocia, or perineal lacerations.[11] All scientific studies published in the medical literature about the best way to 'manage' particular obstetric situations or particular phases of labor are conducted in environments where the fetus ejection reflex is ignored and inhibited. And no fetus ejection reflex occurs when the birth process is 'managed'.

A powerful hormonal flow

We cannot interpret the fetus ejection reflex in the current scientific context without referring to the complex interactions between the components of the powerful hormonal flow involved in such a short and critical event: oxytocin, endorphins, prolactin, vasopressin, hormones of the adrenaline family, probably melatonin, etc... It is particularly useful, from a practical perspective, to understand the complexity of the effects of hormones of the adrenaline family, as well as the evolutionary advantages of such complexity.

When we refer to the effects of 'adrenaline', we must first emphasize that the term 'adrenaline' is usually a convenient simplified and fast way to refer to the 'hormones of the adrenaline family' (which are otherwise known as 'catecholamines'). In reality there is always a mixture of adrenaline and noradrenaline, and the properties of these two substances are not entirely similar. Either one of them may dominate the other, depending on the situation. However, in general, it is not essential to be aware of these subtleties and the broad definition and meaning of 'adrenaline' may be sufficient. It is often sufficient to know that 'adrenaline' is a hormone which mammals release in emergency situations, particularly when they are scared, when they feel observed, and when they are cold. It is important to understand that, in general, 'adrenaline' inhibits the release of oxytocin, the key hormone during the period surrounding birth. Oxytocin is actually the key hormone since it plays an important mechanical role in inducing and maintaining effective uterine contractions necessary for the birth of the baby and the delivery of the placenta, and because it is the main 'love hormone'. It is also important in practice to realize how contagious the release of 'adrenaline' is among mammals in general. When a member of a group has perceived possible danger, the changes in its hormonal balance send out subtle warning messages. It is the same amongst humans: a woman cannot give birth if there is a person nearby releasing 'adrenaline'.

Being aware of the adrenaline-oxytocin antagonism leads us to explain that 'adrenaline' is the 'brake' that postpones all episodes of the sexual life of mammals when the survival of individuals is threatened and when the priority is to have energy available to fight or flee.[9,10] This is the case, for example, of a female in the jungle who has perceived the presence of a predator: she cannot give birth as long as she does not feel secure. Understanding the adrenaline-oxytocin antagonism also helps us to analyze the basic mammalian needs of a laboring woman: she needs to feel secure, without feeling observed, in a place which is sufficiently warm.

When exploring and rediscovering the ultimate steps of the birth ladder, we must remember that the concept of adrenaline-oxytocin antagonism is a convenient simplification. In reality one cannot completely ignore the complexity of the effects of the hormones of the adrenaline family during the minutes surrounding birth.

The complexity of these effects is easy to anticipate since it is affected by the ratio of adrenaline to noradrenaline, and since there are two kinds of cells that are sensitive to adrenaline in the uterus. When 'beta receptors' are involved, hormones of the adrenaline family tend to restrain or hinder the activity of the uterine muscle. This seems to be the dominant effect during the first, passive stage of labor. The point is that there are also 'alpha receptors' which have, by contrast, stimulating effects on the uterine muscle. They seem to be involved when the dominant component of catecholamines is noradrenaline.[11,12] This is how we can interpret the transitory and paradoxically stimulating effects of hormones of the adrenaline family during a fast and powerful fetus ejection reflex.

This transitory stimulating effect of hormones of the adrenaline family during the fetus ejection reflex is the key to interpreting some puzzling clinical observations. The word 'reflex' first recommended itself to me in very special circumstances. It was in the 1970s, at a time when the media had not yet heard of our approach in the Pithiviers hospital, which often involved replacing drugs during labor with an alternative. Many women had a birthing pool at their disposal, which they could use without having been influenced by what they had read. They could behave in a spontaneous way, since they were not committed to a birth plan. Of course, in the case of a difficult first stage our primary objective was to make contractions more effective by reducing the level of 'adrenaline' through maternal immersion in water at body temperature. Unexpectedly, we observed that often in this environment labor stopped progressing when the baby was not far away from birth.[13] This is the time when many women leave a bath or birthing pool spontaneously. As soon as they return to a cool atmosphere it is as if the different ambient temperature triggers some major contractions and delivery is then fast. This is typical when goose bumps and other symptoms of a surge of adrenaline are obviously compatible with strong and efficient contractions. It is in such circumstances that I found the term 'fetus ejection reflex' relevant to human beings as well. A rapid expulsive stage of delivery triggered by fear is another example of a paradoxical situation in which efficient contractions seem to be associated with increased levels of 'adrenaline'. There are countless anecdotes reported by birth attendants, sometimes in extreme circumstances like bombardments or earthquakes. There has also been the well-known practice of saying or doing something frightening as a way of occasionally avoiding the need to use forceps. Besides, anthropological documents suggest that, at a final stage of labor, in some very precise circumstances, fear has been used to trigger the birth.

Not only can we conclude that a fetus ejection reflex is associated with a release of 'adrenaline', but we can also understand that a release of hormones of the adrenaline family can trigger a fetus ejection reflex.

These phenomena have obvious evolutionary advantages. If anything threatening should occur at the beginning of labor, there is an advantage to postponing the birth and being in a state of muscular activity. On the other hand, having passed the point of no return in labor, it is an advantage to give birth as quickly as possible.

The real climax

At the precise moment of birth the top of the ladder is not far away. However, the real climax is reached a little later, when the mother, still on another planet, is discovering her newborn baby. This is another reason why the orgasmic/ecstatic state associated with childbirth has been ignored in all cultural milieus until recently. It is easy to abruptly interrupt an orgasmic state. As soon as a baby is born, there is always an irrational need for activity around, either the need to talk or the need to do something. This need for activity has been ritualized in many societies and what most of these societies have in common is that they disregard the mother's need for privacy. The deep-rooted belief that the presence of a specialized person is the basic need of laboring women and newborn babies is another reason why the birth climax cannot be understood. In our societies unassisted deliveries occur occasionally, by accident. This is more often than not the case of fast births. Either the midwife could not arrive in time, or the mother could not reach the hospital in time. Because such births are easy, one might anticipate that it is an opportunity for some women to reach a real climax. It is not so in most cases, because of the cultural conditioning that a woman is unable to give birth by herself. For example if the husband/partner is around, he is usually in a state of panic, wondering what he must do and who will 'deliver the baby', and who will cut the cord.

Anecdotal reports confirm how critical these very first minutes are and this is easily interpreted in scientific terms. An accumulation of data confirms the spectacular hormonal upheaval during the minutes before and after birth. The team headed by Kerstin Uvnäs-Moberg have demonstrated that just after giving birth a mother has the capacity to reach a peak of oxytocin that is still higher than for the delivery itself.[14] We can therefore reasonably assume that the highest peak of love hormone a woman has the capacity to release in her whole life is immediately after a birth. This peak of oxytocin is vital since it is necessary for a safe delivery of the placenta with minimum blood loss, and also because oxytocin is the main love hormone. It is undoubtedly associated with high levels of natural morphine and prolactin. Noting that, according to Regina Lederman[15], the level of 'adrenaline' can return to normal as early as three minutes after birth, we can assume that a human mother has a hormonal experience which is similar to that of an orgasm.

While, for many obvious reasons, most practitioners cannot easily understand what the fetus ejection reflex is, they have usually heard of the Ferguson reflex, which was described as early as 1941. Working with anesthetized rabbits, Ferguson found that uterine contractions were induced by vaginal dilatation.[16] The Ferguson reflex is different from the fetus ejection reflex because it does not take into account the paramount importance of environmental factors in the birth process. It just takes into account the effects of local vaginal stimulations among non-human mammals.

By combining recent scientific data and anecdotes about births in exceptionally rare conditions of privacy and security, we can conclude that the human mammal has been programmed to give birth in an ecstatic/orgasmic state, keeping in mind that the release of oxytocin – 'the shy hormone' – is highly dependent on environmental factors. The term 'shy hormone' is a significant example of a term coined by the London doula Liliana Lammers. In the particular case of the minutes following birth, the 'shy hormone' can appear on the condition that the place is warm enough, and on the condition that the mother is not distracted at all when discovering her newborn baby through skin-to-skin contact, eye-to-eye contact, and also via her sense of smell.

From a practical perspective we are now in a position to present authentic midwifery as the art of creating the conditions for a fetus ejection reflex.

3

THE TURNING POINT OF THE 70s

Once, around 1970, I was operating on an elderly woman who had advanced stomach cancer. Since I was busy in the operating room, I was not available to discuss a case of a breech birth with the midwife on duty. This anecdote helped me to realize how vital was the preoccupation of the lonely midwife, compared with the activities of a whole surgical team. When I arrived at the Pithiviers state hospital in 1962, the small midwifery unit was still a sort of enclave attached to the surgical unit. It was large enough to meet local demand and I was comfortable with the situation. In spite of my interest in the evolution of surgical techniques, I also needed opportunities to improve my understanding of human nature in general. Being occasionally involved in the emergence of life was a way to satisfy this need.

A personal turning point

As a result of my ongoing interests and the circumstances within which I was working, I became more and more convinced of the importance of the environment when a woman gives birth. Although it was impossible at that time to discuss such issues with anybody, I tacitly decided to rely on young colleagues to reduce my surgical activity and to spend more time and energy reconsidering which factors might make birth easier or more difficult and which factors might facilitate interaction between mother and newborn baby. The ultimate outcome was that we gradually brought 'home' into the hospital itself. We did this by inviting pregnant women to come and sing together around the piano as a way of making them familiar with both the place and the members of the staff, by designing a small home-like birthing room, and also by reconsidering many other aspects of our practice.[1,2] The objective effect of these dramatic changes was to make our hospital unit extremely popular: we went from having about 200 births a year in 1962 to 1,000 births in a single year in 1977.

In retrospect, the turning point in my own career in the 1970s can be seen as part of the major turning point in the history of childbirth, which started simultaneously in that decade in different parts of the world. It is as if a new awareness was bound to develop at a time when the birthing environment was being altered to an absurd degree.

The socialization of childbirth

In order to analyze the nature and timing of this historical turning point, we must first realize through a fast overview how, and at which point, all societies for thousands of years have disturbed the physiological processes occurring in the perinatal period (the period surrounding birth). In every given society multiple beliefs and rituals usually complete and reinforce the effects of one another.

Modifying the woman's anatomy through ritual genital mutilations is an easily explained method of interference. Female genital mutilations have been observed in Africa, in parts of the near East, in aboriginal Australia, in parts of Oceania and in the Amazon Basin.[3] Today, according to World Health Organization estimates, over 100 million women are affected by this practice. Such interventions always leave a certain amount of inelastic scar tissue. Infibulation, or 'Pharaonic circumcision', is undoubtedly the most invasive procedure. It involves cutting off the whole clitoris, the whole of the labia minora and the adjacent parts of the labia majora and stitching the two sides of the vulva together, so as to leave a small opening for urination and menstruation. This causes prolonged labor and a birth attendant is needed to cut through the soft tissues for the purpose of enlarging the passage. This is one method amongst many others of cultivating a cultural conditioning which suggests that a woman is unable to give birth without the help of an attendant.

For obvious reasons it is difficult to obtain precise information on how women gave birth in preliterate societies. However, we must constantly bear in mind that, from a physiological perspective, there are only two obligatory actors in the birth drama: the mother and the baby. The presence at birth of a 'third person' cannot be considered a basic need. There has been a phase in the history of humanity when women used to isolate themselves when giving birth, like all mammals. This is confirmed by a great diversity of documents, such as films among the Eipos in New Guinea[4], written documents about the !Kung San and other pre-agricultural societies[5], and word-of-mouth reports from Amazonian ethnic groups transmitted in particular by the Brazilian midwife anthropologist Heloisa Lessa. The concept of a birth attendant is more recent than is commonly believed, although a mother or mother figure was probably around when a woman was giving birth in primitive societies. This was mostly to protect the privacy of the birthing woman against the presence of wandering men or animals. No doubt this is how midwifery began.

Everywhere in the world there has been a tendency to dramatically alter the original role of the birth attendant, to deny the birthing woman's need for privacy and to socialize childbirth. More often than not, the midwife has become an agent of the cultural milieu, transmitting its specific beliefs and rituals. In many non-industrial societies, the birth attendant is an authoritarian guide who tries to actively influence a woman's labor by manipulating, kneading or manually dilating the cervix, for example. In one way and another, her aim is often to try to speed up the process of birth.[6]

The phase of labor which is disturbed most profoundly by all societies is the short phase between the birth of the baby and the delivery of the placenta. We might even claim that all societies make impossible the interaction between mother and newborn baby just after the birth. It would take volumes to review all the invasive perinatal beliefs and rituals which have been reported in a great diversity of cultures. As early as 1884 *Labor Among Primitive Peoples* by George Engelmann provided an impressive catalogue of the one thousand and one ways of interfering with the first contact between mother and newborn baby. It described beliefs and rituals occurring in hundreds of ethnic groups on all five continents.[7]

The most universal and intriguing way of interfering with mother-baby contact is simply to promote the belief that colostrum is tainted or harmful to the baby, that it is even a substance which needs to be expressed and discarded.[8] Let us recall that, according to modern biological sciences, colostrum – the thick substance available immediately after the birth – is precious. Let us also recall the newborn baby's ability to search for the nipple and to find it as early as the first hour after the birth. The negative attitude towards colostrum implies that, immediately after the birth, a baby must be in the arms of another person, rather than with his or her own mother. This is the origin of a widespread deep-rooted ritual, which is to rush to cut the cord.[9] Several beliefs and rituals can be seen as part of the same interference, all of them reinforcing each other. For example in some ethnic groups in Benin, West Africa, people transmit the belief that the mother must not look at the baby's eyes during the day following birth, because this might cause 'bad spirits' to enter the baby's body. According to Sobonfu Somé, 'the keeper of rituals', in the Tagara tribe in Burkina Faso when a woman is in labor the young children of the community wait nearby and as soon as they hear the baby's first cry, they all rush to the birthplace, shouting to 'welcome' the baby.[10] What a powerful way to abruptly interrupt the vital peak of oxytocin, which has also been called the 'shy hormone'! Many other rituals can disturb the first contact between mother and baby, typical examples including weighing the baby, bathing, rubbing, tight swaddling, foot binding, 'smoking' the baby, piercing the ears of the little girls and opening the doors in cold countries.

It is noticeable that several variants of the same ritual have been observed in places as far apart as New Guinea and Brazil. Margaret Mead has provided detailed reports of childbirth among the mountain dwelling Arapesh in New Guinea.[11] While his wife is in labor, the father waits within earshot until the sex is determined. When he is informed of the sex of the baby, he laconically answers: 'Wash it' or 'Do not wash it', which means that the child is or is not to be brought up. This clearly indicates that the baby is in the hands of the midwife, who is herself at the service of the father. Among the Myky from Mato Grosso, in Brazil, the mother is not authorized to touch the baby as long as the spiritual leader has not yet confirmed that this particular baby should survive. Among ethnic groups in Amazonia, it is only after receiving permission from the godfather, who will be wearing his ceremonial clothes, that the mother can take care of her baby.

This is a relatively small sample of available data regarding widespread beliefs and rituals. Man's potential for meddling in the newborn baby's relationship with his or her mother – in other words man's capacity to hinder or interrupt any sort of ecstatic-orgasmic state near the top of the birth ladder – is enormous.

When a medical institution takes control

Up until the twentieth century shamanic and religious institutions played an important role in the control of childbirth (as well as other aspects of a person's life). This role was indirect and the role of the medical institution specifically also remained indirect for a long time, mostly via the education of midwives. Socialization via the medical institution has been an important step in the history of childbirth because it gradually made control by the cultural milieu more direct. In most societies women had always been successful in protecting themselves against the presence of men, including medical men, during labor. This point is eloquently illustrated by certain anecdotes. In one case in the eighteenth century, for example, a doctor in Hamburg disguised himself as a woman so he could watch a birth. He was discovered, condemned to death and burnt alive. From the beginning of the twentieth century onwards, a great number of technical, scientific and pharmacological advances dramatically strengthened the power of the medical institution. The control of childbirth by an originally male institution became more and more direct and powerful.

An unprecedented and sophisticated form of culturally controlled childbirth suddenly appeared in the 1950s: the transmission of scientific theories. It became fashionable to teach women how to give birth, and particularly how to breathe during labor and delivery. In 1949 the neuro-psychiatrist Velvovski, a disciple of Pavlov, created the Russian 'psychoprophylactic method', which aimed to eliminate the pain of childbirth. The French obstetrician Lamaze introduced this method into Western countries. In the USA it became known as the 'Lamaze Method'. It was based on the concept of conditioned reflexes. Its main theoretical basis was that the pain of labor is not physiological, but reflex-conditioned and therefore cultural. The promoters of this method had understood that conditioned reflexes are related to the activity of the neocortex (the seat of all inhibitions), but they had not understood the solution Nature had found to overcome difficulties in childbirth... They had not understood that a reduction of the activity of the neocortex is the most important aspect of birth physiology among humans. They had not understood that a woman in labor must be protected from any sort of neocortical stimulation and that she must forget what she learned. Instead they thought that pregnant women needed be reconditioned through education and that laboring women needed to be guided via the use of language.

Directly or indirectly, the influence of this method based on the work of theorists has been – and still is – enormous all over the world. Instead of identifying the basic needs of women in labor in order to facilitate labor and delivery and to reduce the needs for drugs and intervention, the focus in recent decades has been on the elimination of pain and fear via non-pharmacological 'methods'. The ambition of some obstetricians was to attach their name to such 'methods', in the same way that practitioners of previous generations were proud to give their name to different kinds of forceps. New actors entered the birth territory: helpers, guides, 'coaches', physiotherapists, psychologists and, in French, 'monitrices d'accouchement sans douleur' (which means 'monitors of pain-free confinement')... The conditioning of new generations of mothers was that women were not able to give birth without the guidance of an expert. The word 'privacy' was ignored, just as what I call 'authentic midwifery' was ignored. The socialization of childbirth had entered a new phase in its long history.

All these phenomena developed side by side at such a high speed after the Second World War that in the 1970s the birth environment had reached an extreme and unprecedented degree of masculinization. First the number of doctors – mostly male doctors – who specialized in obstetrics had increased to such a point that many obstetricians had enough time to become involved in every single birth which took place in their facilities, even the easiest ones. At the same time, other specialized doctors, particularly anesthetists and pediatricians, were more and more visible in the delivery rooms and it was around 1970 that in many countries the doctrine of the participation of the baby's father at birth was established. If we add that the delivery rooms were then invaded by electronic machines and that high technology may be considered a male symbol, we must realize that, for the first time in the history of humanity, women were supposed to have their babies in a male environment.

It is difficult to give a definition of terms such as 'sacredness' and some might even claim that it is impossible to define. When the definition of a term is too difficult it is often relevant to refer to its opposite; so if I personally had to explain what a sacred place is I would bypass the difficulties by presenting a delivery room of the 1970s as the opposite. At that time an absurd point had been reached and it prompted people to start realizing the importance of environmental factors on the way women give birth and babies are born. It was the perfect time for a new awareness to emerge.

Scattered local initiatives

At the very time when an absurd point had been reached, several isolated constructive initiatives were the sudden expression of an emerging new consciousness in several parts of the industrialized world. For example, the Santa Cruz Birth Center was opened in 1972, while several Californian lay midwives were reviving the concept of home birth. At the same time a group of San Francisco hippies left the west coast 'to invent a new lifestyle'. They eventually created 'The Farm' community in Tennessee. This is how Ina May Gaskin and other mothers in the same group became midwives. It was also in the 1970s that the New York Maternity Center opened. Meanwhile, in the context of a French state hospital, we were still trying to bring the home into the hospital, as we've already noted, by doing things like arranging singing sessions around the piano, creating 'home-like birthing rooms' and using birthing pools to replace drugs. (Actually, we cannot mention our birthing pools in Pithiviers without also noting that at the same time in Moscow, Igor Tcharkosky – originally a swimming instructor – was challenging the Russian medical system by starting the swimming training of babies during semi-clandestine home births.)

Secondary links were established between these local isolated initiatives. For example, several Californian lay midwives, such as Mary Jackson from Santa Barbara, spent some time in our maternity unit at Pithiviers so as to confirm what they had learned through their own experience. In the same way, after visiting me the famous diver Jacques Mayol 'discovered' Igor Tcharkosky in Moscow and established links between us. Furthermore, several women suddenly took the initiative to write books which were inspired by their experience as mothers. While British women were reading *The Experience of Childbirth* by Sheila Kitzinger, in 1970s California Suzanne Arms was writing her book *Immaculate Deception*. The main characteristic of books published at that time was their novelty in terms of content and style. Ina May Gaskin's *Spiritual Midwifery* cannot be compared with any other previously published book: 'The Farm', as a birthing place in the countryside in Tennessee represented a perfect antithesis to a modern hospital obstetrics department. It is significant that at the same time Frederick Leboyer wrote *Birth Without Violence,* not as a doctor, but as a man who had re-experienced his own birth through a therapy derived from Indian traditions.

This new generation of books focusing on childbirth should also be presented in the framework of the beginnings of a sort of cultural revolution that has some historical links with the student rebellions of the late 1960s in Paris and California, in particular. All aspects of lifestyle in affluent societies were reconsidered and institutions were scrutinized, criticized, and even blamed or condemned. In his book *Medical Nemesis* (published in 1974) Ivan Illich condemned the expropriation of health by exploring the various supposed aims of the medical institution (the suppression of pain, the eradication of diseases and the struggle against death). However, although he examined the medicalization of old age and death in some detail, he did not consider the medicalization of childbirth at all. This was the reason for my book *Bien Naitre*, published in 1976 (in English it became 'Entering the World'). Among this new generation of books that participated in the induction of a new awareness we must also include *The Primal Scream,* which was published by Arthur Janov in 1970. For the first time the general public was given an opportunity to realize that the way we are born might have lifelong consequences.

The scientific context of the 1970s

Decisive scientific advances accompanied and even supported this new awareness. Inversely research was probably to some extent influenced by the cultural context. In 1973 Karl von Frisch, Konrad Lorenz, and Nikolaas Tinbergen shared the Nobel Prize in physiology and medicine; we had learned from them that among all mammals there is immediately after birth a short period of time which will never occur again and which is critical for mother-baby attachment. The work of these ethologists (and other ethologists, particularly Harlow) prompted practitioners such as Bowlby in the UK and Marshall Klaus and John Kennell in the USA to test 'attachment theory' among humans.

It was also in the 1970s that we heard about a biological system called 'the system of prostaglandins' and learnt about its crucial role in birth physiology. In the same decade the natural opiates called 'endorphins' were discovered, the first experiments demonstrating the behavioural effects of oxytocin were conducted and Regina Lederman studied the inhibitory effect of adrenaline on the birth process.

In such a scientific and cultural climate we were beginning to observe – as ethologists would have done – how mother and newborn baby interacted in the minutes following birth when the physiological processes had been disturbed as little as possible. As a result, new topics of interest emerged: we realized the importance of the first skin-to-skin contact between mother and baby, the first eye-to-eye contact between mother and newborn and also the importance of the mother's and baby's sense of smell during these crucial minutes. We began to understand that human babies have been programmed to express the 'rooting reflex' and therefore to find the nipple during the hour following birth,[12,13,14] at the very time when the mother is still in a state of special hormonal balance and in an instinctive state which means that she is able to perfectly coordinate her own behavior with that of her baby.

Our overview of how cultural milieus dramatically disturb the physiological processes of birth has been necessary to clarify the significance of the 1970s as a turning point. There are obstacles to the spreading of the emerging new awareness. Technical advances which directly govern the practices of modern obstetrics and midwifery become established quickly, while scientific and conceptual advances spread out slowly. For example the simplified technique of the cesarean operation, which was recently developed by Michael Stark, is now well known and even practiced on the five continents, while most practitioners still know very little about the different aspects of the 'scientification of love', including the behavioral effects of oxytocin. However, in spite of powerful barriers after thousands of years of culturally controlled childbirth, it is noticeable that there is already in every country a tiny core of people who are ready to formulate radically new questions.

From now on, all questions regarding orgasmic states and their functions are bound to refer to the top of the 'birth ladder' – a situation unanticipated some decades ago, even perhaps by Wilhelm Reich.

4

MEN ALSO HAVE ORGASMS

If we look at the genital ladder, we inevitably have to consider the male sex as well. However, in order to appreciate the similarities between the birth ladder and the genital ladder, we will first consider the genital orgasmic states women experience.

Before penetrating the complexity of human behavior and interpreting the vulnerability of human beings in all episodes of their sexual lives, we will look at our mammalian roots. Our study of the fetus ejection reflex gave us an opportunity to present *Homo sapiens* as a mammal with a huge and powerful 'new brain'. As we have already noted, when our neocortex manages to become less active, we become more similar to mammals, such as mice or rats. In other words, when our neocortex is suppressed our basic mammalian being expresses itself more freely in behavioral terms.

* * *

The road from simplicity towards complexity

This is why, before considering women's orgasms, we will refer to studies using rodents (in this case rats) to understand basic female mating behavior. This will help us to appreciate the similarities between the fetus ejection reflex and the female mating reflexes.

Komisaruk and Larsson demonstrated that when a probe is inserted into a rat's vagina and pressed gently against the cervix the rat is immobilized (her legs become rigidly extended and her abdominal muscles tense).[1] This is exactly the female rat response during mating. If the strength of the immobilization is challenged by pinching a hind paw or the tail with toothed forceps, the normally immediate leg withdrawal response is completely blocked. Komisaruk and his colleagues found that when human women use vaginal self-stimulation in laboratory studies leg withdrawal is inhibited during toe pinching in the same way.[2] This illustration shows how a good knowledge of basic mammalian behavior can be useful as a guide to research on humans.

Studies among rats should also guide the research regarding the similarities between mating behavior and the fetus ejection reflex. These similarities are striking where non-human mammals are concerned. Leg extension, immobilization, and abdominal muscle tensing also occur during the fetus ejection reflex among rats, which is the other occasion when the female receives vaginal and cervical stimulation naturally. Leg extension facilitates the emergence of the pups from the vagina, while the abdominal muscle tensing enables ejection to occur; this is confirmed by the finding that blocking the induced muscle contraction by cutting the pelvic nerves prevents delivery of the pups.[3]

Furthermore, the brain regions which are activated during mating and vaginal and cervical stimulation have been identified among rats. This sort of research is possible today by making visible a specific protein produced in a neuron when stimulated (the 'c-fos method'). We can conclude that one of the most active brain structures during mating is the 'paraventricular nucleus of the hypothalamus' (commonly called PVN).[4] This is noticeable since the PVN neurons secrete oxytocin, which is stored in the posterior pituitary gland before being released into the general bloodstream. The nucleus accumbens, important for the local release of dopamine, is also activated during mating.[5] In other words the dopaminergic 'reward' system is activated during mating.

Introducing uni-orgasmic sex

While we have been investigating the birth ladder, the fetus ejection reflex, and basic female mammalian mating behavior, we have been focusing on physiological processes in one gender only. This has been the necessary step in order to understand how artificial it is to consider the female response during sexual intercourse in isolation from the act of giving birth. The similarities are striking from an objective perspective in terms of behavioral and neurohormonal responses. They are also striking from a subjective perspective: women who had the opportunity to reach the top of the birth ladder use the words 'ecstatic' and 'orgasmic'. I have heard women comparing their transcendental emotional state when giving birth and interacting with their newborn babies with occasional cosmic consciousness they have experienced during sexual intercourse... which is what Helene Deutsch, as a free woman, dared to do as early as 1924.[6]

However, when considering the genital ladder we also have to raise some preliminary questions about the similarities and the differences between male and female orgasms.

Vance and Wagner performed an ingenious controlled study among college students in order to compare male and female orgasms from a subjective perspective.[7] Male and female students wrote descriptions of their own orgasms, and a group of judges tried to guess which descriptions were written by men and which by women. The judges were female and male obstetrician-gynecologists, psychologists and medical students. Before submitting the descriptions to the judges, the researchers substituted gender-neutral words for specific words in the descriptions (for example 'genitalia' for 'penis' or 'vagina'). After statistical analysis, the authors concluded that 'individuals are unable to distinguish the sex of a person from that person's written description of his or her orgasm… Furthermore, neither sex was more adept at recognizing characteristics in descriptions of orgasm that would serve as a basis for sex discrimination…'

In spite of similarities between men and women regarding their descriptions of subjective experiences, there are crucial objective differences. The main one is that women can experience multiple orgasms. This means that orgasms can occur in succession, without loss of sexual arousal in between. In men, on the other hand, the sperm ejection reflex (or 'ejaculatory orgasm') initiates a refractory period. During this 'resolution phase', which can last several hours, men cannot achieve another erection or even receive further stimulation because the penis is too sensitive to touch.

Sensations conveyed by genital nerves

The similarities between men and women are also more striking than the differences when considering the division of labor among genital sensory nerves. The pudendal nerves convey orgasm-producing stimulations from the clitoris in women and from the penis and the scrotum in men. The hypogastric nerves convey stimulations from the cervix and the uterus in women and from the testes and prostate in men. The pelvic nerves convey stimulations from the vagina, the cervix, the bladder and the rectum. Furthermore the vagus nerves might convey stimulations from the cervix and the uterus.[2]

It is easier to dissociate the effects of these different nerve stimulations among women than among men. Several studies provide evidence for the notion that direct stimulation of the vagina or cervix in the absence of direct clitoral stimulation can generate an orgasm. Furthermore, women describe the quality of orgasms resulting from vaginal stimulation as different from orgasms induced only by clitoral stimulation.[8] While stimulating the clitoris, the vagina or the cervix separately can produce orgasms, the combined stimulation of all three regions has an additive effect, producing more encompassing orgasms, or what is described as 'blended orgasm'.[9] Interestingly, it is also worth noting that among humans, an orgasm can be reached without genital stimulation. In some circumstances, psychological stimulation alone can be sufficient. Finally, it is worth emphasizing that all these genital sensory nerves reach the same brain structures, particularly the paraventricular nucleus of the hypothalamus (the PVN), a cluster of neurons in the hypothalamus which are the major source of oxytocin in the body.

Messages conveyed by oxytocin

The well-documented role of oxytocin during sexual arousal and orgasm serves to remind us how artificial it is to dif-
ferentiate between the nervous system and the endocrine
system. Oxytocin can act as a neurotransmitter (a messenger between neurons) at different levels of the nervous system. It can also act as a conventional hormone since it can
be released directly into the blood stream from neurons in
the brain. The paramount importance of oxytocin also
serves to remind us of the many similarities between male
and female orgasms.

As early as 1987 a team from Stanford University headed
by Marie Carmichael published a study in which oxytocin
levels among men and women during masturbation and
orgasm were measured continuously via indwelling venous
catheters.[10] The subject could press a signal to indicate the
start and finish of orgasm/ejaculation. The shapes of the
graphs were similar between men and women. However it
is noticeable that the levels during self-stimulation before
orgasm were higher among women. They were also higher
among women during orgasm, and multi-orgasmic women
reached a higher peak during the second orgasm. In another study the same team found a positive correlation, among
both men and women, between oxytocin levels and the
intensity, but not the duration, of orgasmic contractions.[11]
For multi-orgasmic women the amount of the increase of
oxytocin level also related to the subjective report about
orgasm intensity.

During any episode of our reproductive life, oxytocin has
both behavioral and mechanical effects. During female
orgasm the immediate effect of the release of oxytocin is to

induce uterine contractions which help to transport the sperm towards the egg. This was demonstrated in 1961 by two American surgeons during a gynecological operation.[12] Before making the abdominal incision they introduced particles of carbon into the woman's vagina near to the cervix and simultaneously administered an injection of oxytocin. They later found particles of carbon in the woman's fallopian tubes. The occurrence of uterine contractions during orgasm in pregnant and non-pregnant women has been confirmed by further studies among non-pregnant and pregnant women.[13,14] Among men, during the sperm ejection reflex, the release of oxytocin helps to induce contractions of the prostate and seminal vesicles.[15] The term 'sperm ejection reflex' is convenient as a way to remind us that not only are the same hormones involved in different episodes of sexual life, but also that the same patterns are reproduced. Using this term serves to remind us of the similarities this reflex has with the 'fetus ejection reflex' and the 'milk ejection reflex'.

Natural morphines

Although it is difficult to demonstrate this directly in humans, it is widely accepted that both partners release high levels of endorphins during orgasm. This has been found to be the case in laboratory animals such as mice, rats, rabbits, dogs, monkeys, and chimpanzees, and we can assume the same must be true for human beings.[16] Beta endorphin levels in the blood of male hamsters after their fifth ejaculation were found to be 86 times higher than those of control animals.

The importance of the system of endorphins has been

confirmed among humans by studies which take into account interactions between oxytocin and endorphin systems. British researchers observed the effects of naloxone on men while they were experiencing an orgasm (this drug blocks the effects of morphine-like substances). Oxytocin levels did not increase among men who were injected with naloxone, but they increased to 362% of baseline values at orgasm with a placebo.[17] Furthermore, a decrease in the level of subjective arousal and pleasure at orgasm was noted after injection with naloxone. This study is a convincing demonstration of the importance of the system of endorphins during orgasm. Since endorphins are the main releasers of prolactin, the paramount role of the system of endorphins during orgasm is also suggested by the concordant results of all studies which detected high levels of prolactin immediately after male and female orgasms.[18,19,20,21] Finally, brain-imaging experiments have revealed activation of the same zones, particularly the ventral tegmental area, as well as the deactivation of the amygdala, during both the sperm ejection reflex and a heroin rush.[33]

The release of endorphins as natural painkillers easily explains the analgesic effect of orgasms. A person's pain threshold has been measured as the force at which a gradually increasing compression of the fingers becomes painful.[22,23,24] In experiments, continuously maintained pressure stimulation on the anterior vaginal wall produced a more than 50 percent increase in the pain threshold, while comparable pressure stimulation of the posterior vaginal wall had no significant effect. In another study, when participants were asked to use vaginal self-stimulation in a way that felt pleasurable, significant analgesia was elicited by stimulating all the genital regions. The greatest increase in pain threshold occurred when self-stimulation resulted in orgasm, although it is interesting to note that the increased pain threshold was not associated with a change in touch thresholds, measured as sensitivity to gentle touch stimulation on the back of the hand. These findings indicate that vaginal self-stimulation produces analgesia rather than anesthesia and they certainly suggest an opiate effect. Migraine sufferers confirm the analgesic effect of orgasm. In a study of 83 women who suffered migraine, orgasm resulted in at least some relief for more than 50 percent of subjects.[25]

The adrenaline family

The complexity of the effects of the hormones of the adrenaline family during sexual arousal and genital orgasms leads us once more to emphasize the similarities between the 'birth ladder' and the 'genital ladder'. Just as the first phase of labor and the fetus ejection reflex must be conceptualized as distinct and sequential phases, so must sexual arousal and genital orgasm also be contrasted. Just as there are two sorts of uterine receptors to hormones of the adrenaline family involved in the birth process, there are also alpha and beta-adrenergic receptors in the penis, the clitoris and the vagina. Just as hormones of the adrenaline family inhibit the first phase of labor, so do these hormones also play a role in inhibiting sexual arousal among men and women, in maintaining the penis in a flaccid state, and in producing detumescence after the sperm ejection reflex.[26, 27] Just as females cannot give birth if there is a predator around, couples can also not make love in life-threatening situations. Finally, just as the fetus ejection reflex is associated with high levels of hormones of the adrenaline family, involving alpha-receptors in particular, so also are orgasms of genital sexuality associated with high levels of noradrenaline, involving alpha-receptors specifically.

Messages conveyed by other informational substances

At the current time terms such as hormones, the endocrine system, the nervous system and the immune system are confusing, since certain substances sometimes behave as conventional hormones do and sometimes as neurotransmitters, and since certain messengers can be released either by nerve cells, or by cells with immune actions, or even by endocrine glands. This is why we shall refer to these messengers as 'ligands', or 'informational substances'.

Our objective is not to offer a comprehensive review of all the studies in progress regarding the roles of countless other informational substances involved in orgasmic states: androgens, estrogens, progesterone, vasopressin, cortisol, histamine, gamma-aminobutyric acid, acetylcholine, etc. We will mention the importance of studies regarding just two modulators of sexual behavior: dopamine and serotonin. Dopamine tends to facilitate sexual activity among mammals, birds and reptiles. It is one of the components of the 'reward system', alongside oxytocin and endorphins. Serotonin, on the other hand, acts as a 'brake' on sexual behavior. We must also mention the many recent studies regarding the release of nitric oxide by the nerves that reach the penis. The importance of such studies are easily understood when one knows that nitric oxide plays an indirect role in the relaxation of the smooth muscles which control the diameters of the small arteries going to the penis, and therefore the local blood flow.

Although it has been the subject of considerable speculation in the popular scientific literature, we shall intentionally pay only a small amount of attention to pheromones, ie to substances excreted externally by the body. Although these pheromones have no obvious odor, the vomeronasal organ in the nose of mammals picks them up so the pheromone system is of paramount importance in the sexual behavior of non-human mammals. When the vomeronasal organ of female mice has been removed, or when female mice have been engineered to lack a gene essential for the function of this organ, these mice act exactly like males: with mounting, pelvic thrusts and even the ultrasound calls males use to attract a mate.[28] Among most humans there is probably the equivalent of a small vomeronasal organ which is a minor contributor to sexual attraction. Karl Grammer made a study of the effects on men of vaginal pheromones known as copulins. His research showed that the male pheromone androsterone, found in underarm sweat, is attractive to women when they are ovulating and at their most fertile.[29] Our current knowledge of the role of pheromones on sexual attractiveness has been reinforced by experiments conducted at the Athena Institute for Women's Wellness Research in Pennsylvania.[30] These experiments tested whether synthesized human pheromones increase the sociosexual behavior of men.

In the age of brain imaging

Our current understanding of hormonal balance during

genital orgasms has been supported by the development of sophisticated brain imaging techniques. With Positron Emission Tomography (PET), for example, it is possible to identify the brain areas which are working hardest by measuring their radioactivity after injecting water labeled with an isotope of oxygen. Functional Magnetic Resonance Imaging (FMR), on the other hand, can show up areas where there is most oxygen. These techniques have rapidly surpassed previous methodologies such as electrical stimulation of the brain and electroencephalography.

Finnish researchers have been the first to demonstrate that during an orgasm the neocortex is at rest, apart from the right prefrontal cortex.[31] They refer to a parallel with an earlier report on hypersexuality in men with a lesion disconnecting the prefrontal cortex from the rest of the brain[32] and to the disinhibited sexuality that may occur after frontal lobotomy, that is to say a partial separation of the frontal lobes from the rest of the brain. All these sophisticated perspectives confirm the obvious and the essential, ie that during any sort of sexual experience, the neocortex is a source of inhibition.

It is not surprising that imaging the brain during orgasm has demonstrated an activation of many deep brain structures, in particular the paraventricular nucleus of the hypothalamus (PVN), which is the source of oxytocin, as well as the nucleus accumbens, the basal ganglia, the insula, the cingulated cortex, and the hippocampus.[2] The Dutch authors of the most sophisticated study of brain imaging during male orgasms confirmed that neocortical activity persists only in a small number of zones (Brodmann areas 7/40, 18, 21, 23, and 47), exclusively on the right side of the brain.[33] A salient and reliable feature of the brain regions involved in orgasm is strong activation of the cerebellum. Since the role of the cerebellum is to regulate muscle tension, this means that orgasm has a total body response.[34] According to the Dutch researchers these findings corroborate the recent notion that the cerebellum plays an important role in emotional processing. Some years later the same team published a similar study of brain imaging during female orgasm. Female orgasm was mainly associated with profound cerebral blood flow decreases in the neocortex, when compared with control conditions (clitoral stimulation without orgasm and imitation of orgasm).[35]

After this overview of the 'genital ladder' following our exploration of the ultimate steps of the 'birth ladder', we will remember the many similarities between the fetus ejection reflex and genital orgasms. It is artificial to study them separately. There are clear similarities between the immediate post orgasmic states following a fetus ejection reflex and an orgasm of genital sexuality. During the hour following birth, when mother and newborn baby are in close skin-to-skin contact and have not yet eliminated the hormones released during the ejection reflex, each of these hormones has a specific role to play – natural morphine being a typical example. Since all opiates have the properties necessary to create states of dependency, it seems obvious that body-to-body contact between two individuals who are under the effects of endorphins can induce the beginning of a co-dependency, or in other words of an attachment. In the same way, after a shared orgasm, both partners are still under the effects of oxytocin, endorphins, prolactin, vasopressin, and noradrenaline, in particular, and this can be the beginning of an attachment that replicates the mother-baby attachment. Similar scenarios are constantly reproduced.

5

FROM GILGAMESH TO
21ST CENTURY AWARENESS

Recently in the history of humanity, at a time when agricultural societies were well established and the domination of nature was already a basic strategy for the survival of most human groups, some groups of people still knew about genital orgasm as a path to transcendence.

Miraculously preserved documents

The Epic of Gilgamesh, which dates from the third millennium BC, was miraculously preserved on clay tablets in Mesopotamia and excavated in the nineteenth century.[1] Enkidu, one of the main characters of the epic, was considered the strongest man in the world. He was sharing the life of wild animals and 'knew nothing of the cultivated lands'. The trappers were scared of him and didn't dare get close to him. However, they wanted to neutralize him, because he was able to help animals avoid traps. The powerful King Gilgamesh advised a trapper on how to overpower this man. He suggested that only a sacred harlot from the

Temple of Love could do it. This is how for 'six days and seven nights' Enkidu and the harlot laid together. While he was lying on her murmuring love she taught him 'the woman's art'. When he was satisfied he went back towards the wild beasts, but when the wild creatures saw him, they fled. So he returned and sat down at the woman's feet and listened intently to what she said: 'Now, Enkidu, you have become like a god…'

There are many lessons to learn from this epic. First we learn that after such an experience Enkidu underwent a miraculous transformation. He became separated from the animal kingdom because of the significant specifically human function of orgasms. We learn that the initiator, the one who had the knowledge and who could teach, was the woman: this suggests that women are better equipped than men to reach transcendent emotional states through sexual experiences. Furthermore, we learn that Enkidu 'became like a god': this suggests that his orgasmic states were a path to transcendence.

Still more recently the Hindu cult of Ectasy also saw orgasmic states as a means of reaching a cosmic state of consciousness. A parable found in a Tantric text, written in Sanskrit two thousand years ago, is highly significant.[2] It is the story of a hermit pilgrim in search of 'The Supreme Truth'. He had been traveling, meditating, fasting, and inflicting unbearable pain upon himself for many years, but he felt he could never reach the Supreme Truth. One day, disillusioned by years of unrewarded effort, he rested in the late afternoon by a river. A female Tantric Master came along, intending to bathe and anoint her body. After listening to the pilgrim's story she seduced him by 'carrying his senses through Tantric pleasures to the state of extremest arousal, wherein he found the centre of power he sought, awaiting him in what he had so long denied himself.' Once more, the teacher was the woman.

Other miraculously preserved documents include the secret gospels, which were hidden since the first century and only discovered by a ploughman in 1945 in Egypt, near Nag Hammadi. In one of the documents, the Gospel of Thomas, in a conversation with his disciple, it is recorded that Jesus said: 'Make the male and the female into a single One... then you'll enter the kingdom'.

Today a new awareness is emerging. More and more women – and even men – refer to concepts such as transcendent sex. It is significant that the book 'Transcendent Sex', subtitled 'when lovemaking opens the veil', was written by a woman.[3]

Just as we had to clarify the significance of the turning point in the history of childbirth which took place in the 1970s, we also need to have an overview of how cultural milieus have dramatically interfered with genital sexuality before the twenty-first century, and to understand the significance of these interferences.

Culturally controlled orgasmic states

For thousands of years, all aspects of sexuality, including genital sexuality, have been highly controlled and organized by cultural milieus. Mating has been institutionalized, and sexual renunciation has often been made a virtue. Countless aspects of universal sexual repression have been documented.

The most spectacular aspect of the imposed renunciation of sexual pleasure is undoubtedly female genital mutilation. Female circumcision (when only the hood of the clitoris is supposed to be removed), clitoridectomy (when the whole clitoris is removed) and infibulation (when labia majora and minora are also cut away with the razor) are specifically and consciously designed to reduce a woman's capacity to obtain sexual pleasure. In ethnic groups where these rituals prevail, a girl who attempts to avoid the operation is socially ostracized. Uncircumcised women are considered 'unclean'. To call a woman 'the uncircumcised one', or a man 'the son of an uncircumcised woman', is an insult of the most extreme proportions.[4] Interestingly, though, despite these large-scale human experiments in reproduction, even after a clitoridectomy or infibulation some women are still able to have strong sexual feelings.[5]

Male genital mutilation is usually less invasive than female mutilation, but is more widespread and has been practiced on all five continents, even in places such as Oceania, the Asian and Pacific islands, and the New World. Incision usually consists of either a simple cut to the foreskin to draw blood, or a complete cutting through the foreskin in a single place to partly expose the glans. In circumcision itself, the foreskin is completely removed. Subincision, which is usually associated with circumcision, was practiced in particular among Australian aborigines; it involves cutting open the urethra on the underside of the penis down almost as far as the scrotum. Phallotomy and castration, other forms of genital mutilation we must also mention, were most often forced upon young boys who, as captured slaves, would supply the 'needs' of the Arab and Turk system. The use of castration or phallotomy as a punishment, by both individuals and by the state, has been institutionalized in many parts of the world, particularly in the Near East.[6]

Through the practice of compulsory genital mutilations

cultural milieus send significant, although discreet, messages to members of their group. One of the messages is that genitalia belong to the community rather than to individuals, which means that their use must follow strict established rules. Another conditioning effect of such rituals is that the genital parts of the body may remain associated with pain rather than pleasure.

Societies have many other subtle ways to control and restrain all aspects of genital sexuality. The choice of mates, in other words the organization of marriages, is the most universal one. Whatever the details of matrimonial arrangements, the wife is usually considered the property of the husband. In many societies men obtain wives only through difficult or extreme means, namely bride-price, bride-wealth, or through the exchange of a female relative. Marriage rules more often than not favor locating the new couple near the male kin of either spouse. In the Old Testament of the Bible, the woman is listed with other chattels: 'Thou shall not covet thy neighbor's house, thou shall not covet thy neighbor's wife, nor his manservant, nor his ox, nor his ass, nor any thing that is thy neighbor's'. As long as the wife is a property, it is not surprising that women's emotional states during sexual union are ignored. However, there are exceptional situations: one of the seven hundred wives who 'belonged' to King Salomon could express her feelings when making love:

> To me, my beloved is like a cachet of myrrh
> Lying between my breasts.
> To me, my lover is like a cluster of henna
> In the en-Gedi vineyards.
> *The Songs of Songs 1:13-14*

Repression of the powerful sexual drive of adolescence and taboos relating to virginity are quasi-universal aspects of general subordination of the child to the adult will, and of the female to the male. In some regions, loss of virginity before marriage may be so 'dishonorable' to the family that the offending girl will be put to death by her own brother or father. In the same way, sexual intercourse between a married person and someone other than his or her spouse is condemned and severely punished in most cultural milieus.

Present-day studies have usually come to the conclusion that self-genital stimulation is a normal phase in the development of human sexual behavior. However in most societies it has been prohibited and associated with guilt, shame, sinfulness and poor health. The deep-rooted cross-cultural beliefs, traditionally transmitted by religious institutions, were highly supported by 'scientific theories' after the eighteenth century. A new step was reached when Tissot, a respected Swiss Professor of Medicine, published in 1760 his famous book about 'onanism'. Tissot included in the concept of onanism masturbation, anal or oral sex, or sex with contraception. According to his calculations, the loss of one ounce of semen has the same consequences as the loss of 40 ounces of blood. Such theories were the basis of his warnings of the dangers of sex, specifically the dangers of sex undertaken for the purpose of pleasure rather than reproduction. The dangers are still greater in the case of female masturbation because, according to Tissot, the fluid of vaginal lubrication is even more precious than male semen since women's nerves are weaker.

Emerging from a long tunnel

After thousands of years of powerful control over genital functions by cultural milieus, it is not surprising that simple natural paths to transcendence have been ignored or stifled. Mystical emotions have been associated, on the contrary, with sexual renunciation, celibacy, and virginity. The most commonly mentioned paths to transcendence have been fasting, illness, pain, chatisty, loneliness, artistic expression, techniques of meditation, shamanic trance, and hallucinogenic plants. The best known and most influential mystics did not consider the transient ecstatic states of orgasms as possible paths to permanent transformation of consciousness, be they male mystics such as Shankara, Ibn Arabi or Meister Eckhart, or even female mystics such as Hildegard of Bingen, Julian of Norwich, Catherine of Siena or Clare of Assisi. It is as if many aspects of human nature had been concealed for thousands of years. It is as if we are now emerging from a long tunnel.

During this long period in the dark it is also not surprising that falling in love has been considered pathological. This is confirmed by the vocabulary used in a great diversity of languages: 'love fever', 'madly in love', 'love foolishness', *amoureux fou, loco(a) de amor*. 'Infatuation' comes from Latin *fatuus*, which means 'foolish'. The concept of *falling* in love is also widespread in Western and Eastern languages. When people fall in love they do not easily accept subordination to strict regulations. The period of infatuation is characterized by a reduced capacity to think rationally. These irrational behaviors and their unpredictable timing are incompatible with the institutionalized control of genital sexuality. Since they shake the very foundations of our societies, they are often deemed pathological.

Is falling in love really pathological?

Today, multiple scientific perspectives suggest that the period of infatuation is a hard-wired human behavioral pattern with probable evolutionary advantages. There are many reasons to believe that romantic love is the sophisticated expression in our species of universal behavioral patterns: mammals and birds regularly express preferences and choices for a certain mate. Data on such animal behavior suggest that a behavioral 'attraction system' is associated with dopaminergic reward pathways. We can see romantic love as a sophisticated form of this attraction system. This has been confirmed by Functional Magnetic Resonance Imaging in a study of seventeen people who were infatuated.[7] Viewing pictures of the beloved person activated the brainstem right ventral tegmental area and right posterodorsal body of the caudate nucleus, which suggests that dopaminergic reward and motivation pathways contribute to the state of infatuation. A previous study with similar brain scanning concluded that a unique network is involved in becoming infatuated.[8]

A hormonal perspective could also conclude that falling in love remains a complex, specific entity. It is likely that diverse neurotransmitters and hormonal agents are involved in specific ways during the process of infatuation. A naturally-occurring amphetamine substance called phenylethylamine (PEA) seems to play a key role in stimulating romantic love.[9] After a time, the brain tends to become less sensitive to the effect of PEA, or the level of

PEA begins to drop: this signals the end of the period of infatuation. Subjects who are in the early romantic phase of a love relationship have a low density of the platelet serotonin transporter.[10] (The serotonin system is known to modulate mood, emotion, sleep, and appetite and thus is implicated in the control of numerous behavioral and physiological functions).

According to an Italian study, testosterone levels become reduced when men are in love, but elevated when women are in love. It therefore seems that the transient hormonal changes associated with the period of infatuation are sex-specific.[11] Another Italian study suggests that raised levels of nerve growth factor are associated with the early stages of romantic love, and that there is a significant positive correlation between these levels and the intensity of romantic love as assessed on a 'passionate love scale'.[12] Some behavioral and emotional features associated with falling in love could be related to raised nerve growth factor levels in the bloodstream.

The concept of infatuation as a hard-wired human behavioral pattern is supported by anthropological studies. It appears that romantic love is universal and not a product of any particular culture. Researchers from the University of Honolulu compared the 'passionate love scales' and the 'companionate love scales' of college students from an individualist culture (USA) and from a collectivist culture (Korea). No cultural difference was found.[13] A survey presented at a session of the American Anthropological Association in 1992 found romantic love described in 147 cultures out of 166. What of the other 19? According to the organisers of the session, it is probable that the anthropologists were simply unable to recognise different variations of romantic behavior confined to these unfamiliar cultures.

We might argue that anthropologists can only study civilized human groups that have established culturally controlled mating. It is well known that infatuation thrives on frustration and flourishes under difficult circumstances. It is also well known that there is a reinforced appeal for an object of desire considered illegal, immoral or at least difficult to obtain. One can therefore hypothesize that the concept of 'forbidden fruit' – a consequence of rules and barriers – provides a breeding ground for the most spectacular aspects of romantic love. It can also conceal the subtle and discreet forms of usually repressed behaviors.

If falling in love is a hard-wired transitory period of reduced rationality during which a conception is likely to occur, one can anticipate that the fashionable concepts of 'prepared conception', 'planned conception', and 'conscious conception' have a limited future – as long as human beings remain endowed with the capacity to fall in love, in other words as long as conception is likely to happen in periods of irrationality. Questions must also be raised about the function of the period of infatuation. The reduced capacity to think rationally during that period might be a way to prepare for the reduced activity of the neocortex while climbing the genital ladder. It might perhaps be a way to prepare an escape from space and time reality up the ultimate steps of the ladder. We might also assume that a woman who has conceived a baby during a period of infatuation is more likely to be joyful while expecting her baby.

Once I was asked to talk at a conference about 'the function of joy in pregnancy'. I had to overcome a major obstacle: although many emotional states have been studied in a scientific way by physiologists, psychologists, epidemiologists and other scientists, the concept of joy has not. Explore scientific and medical databases: the keywords 'anxiety', 'stress', 'depression', 'psychological distress', or 'fear' bring up thousands of references. 'Joy', on the other hand, remains a sterile keyword.

Since it has been said that painters, poets and other artists always precede scientists, I first looked at what we can learn from them about joy. 'The Five Joyful Mysteries' is undoubtedly the most fruitful reference in the field of painting and it is significant that the word 'joy' is associated with the word 'mystery' because 'mystery' has the same root as 'mystic'. In other words, a joyful experience transcends the limits of ordinary experience and takes us into the realms of the mystic. The Annunciation, the Visitation, the Nativity, the Presentation in the Temple and the Finding in the Temple are all events related to the emergence of life. Archetypal joyful experiences are related to maternal love. They are intense responses to rewarding events. We also learn that joy is contagious. After the Annunciation, Mary will share her joy with another mother-to-be. The sacred atmosphere of the Temple is appropriate for the expression of different facets of maternal love.

Poets and musicians are not strangers to joy. The 'Ode to Joy' is now the European anthem, based on the fourth movement of Beethoven's Symphony No 9. One can wonder how the music by Beethoven evokes joy – sudden intermittent series of ascending notes are undoubtedly suggestive of the emergence of life. The original text of the European anthem was the poem written by Friedrich Schiller at the end of the eighteenth century. From the start of the poem, joy is presented as sudden access to the divine: 'Freude, schöner Götterfunken' (Joy, beautiful spark of divinity). The last line of a poem by my own mother about joy ('joie') is also highly significant: 'un grand hymne à la joie évoque le Très-Haut'[14], which can be translated as 'a grand hymn of joy evokes the Almighty'. Poets also symbolically associate joy with the emergence of life. The poem by my mother includes the words 'printemps' (spring), 'oiseau qui chante' (singing birds), 'enfant' (child). The famous song by Charles Trenet is also suggestive of the emergence of life, as it occurs in spring, when the swallows start singing:

'Y'a d'la joie... bonjour, bonjour les hirondelles...'
('There is joy... good morning, good morning swallows...')

After referring to what we can learn from artists, I was at last able to introduce a scientific element to my lecture when I concluded that the study of joyful emotional states could be seen as the antithesis of well-documented states of unhappiness. Our current understanding of the lifelong effects of prenatal exposure to maternal stress hormones can also help us to provide preliminary interpretations of the function of joy in pregnancy. If joy is the opposite of anxiety, depression and psychological distress, we can reasonably assume that it is associated with low levels of cortisol. We can therefore propose that the function of joy in pregnancy is to protect the unborn child against the effects of the harmful stress hormones. Since lasting effects are still detectable in adulthood, we can even understand that joy in pregnancy is necessary to transmit from generation to generation the capacity to be joyful. Let us anticipate that in the near future imaginative scientists will find ways to clarify the role of hormones such as dopamine, serotonin and oxytocin in joyful experiences. Let us also anticipate that the 'scientification of joy' will include the study of unexplored personality traits, such as 'joie de vivre'.

6

THE MILKY WAY

The end of taboos

During a course for nurse-midwives in Brazil the period following birth was the topic of the day. During the discussion, several women started to comment on their own experience of breastfeeding and in particular on their subjective reactions. Some of them used phrases such as 'sexual pleasure', 'sexual arousal', 'ecstatic states' and even 'orgasmic state'. Then a woman suddenly left the room. After the session she came back and explained to the moderator why she had to get out so urgently, overcome by unbearable emotions. About twenty years before, she had decided to stop breastfeeding her one-month-old baby boy simply because she was surprised and distressed each time she experienced intense, orgasmic pleasure during the milk ejection reflex: she felt too guilty and even ashamed to carry on. This course for nurse-midwives was the first opportunity she ever had to become really aware of what happened such a long time before and to express her feelings in words.

There are several lessons to learn from such an anecdote. The main one is that pleasure which can be described as 'sexual' is not exceptionally rare during breastfeeding. Such an anecdote is also a significant reminder of what has been taboo for ages: this nurse had been surprised by her sexual arousal because until recently women did not dare to talk about their emotional states while nursing their babies. This scene is also a reminder that after thousands of years of control, organization and therefore repression of all episodes of human reproductive life, sexual renunciation is usually considered a virtue, while unplanned sexual arousal is morally unacceptable and associated with guilt and shame. Sheila Kitzinger, the mother of five children, offered a perfect inkling of the complexity of these issues in her book *Woman's Experience of Sex*: 'And here, too, reactions vary. One woman delights in the unexpected sexuality of breastfeeding. Another shies away from it because its sexuality confuses her and she feels that two ways in which she uses her body, which ought to be kept completely separate, are getting mixed and confused. This may even bring a sense of moral outrage and revulsion from physical contact with the child, as if the baby is responsible for seducing her'.[1] We must once more save from oblivion the point of view of Helen Deutsch, who was in a position to combine her experience as a mother and medical doctor. During the early 1920s she dared to write: '…the female breast in the act of suckling plays the part of an organ of sexual satisfaction'. Furthermore, she had understood that, in our cultural context, the 'erotogeneity' of the mammary gland frequently leads to feeding difficulties'.[2]

The publication in 1966 by William Masters and Virginia Johnson of a historical title *Human Sexual Response* was undoubtedly an important step in terms of transforming taboos into acceptable topics. The authors were able to openly conclude that for some mothers the nursing experience itself is sexually stimulating enough to carry them to the plateau level of sexual excitement.[3]

I have informally interviewed several of these rare women who gave birth after an authentic fetus ejection reflex. Some of them could compare what they remembered from their experience when at the 'top of the birth ladder' with occasional feelings of sexual arousal or ecstatic states when the baby was at the breast. The similarities were obvious; the differences were in terms of intensity. It is as if the birth ladder, which cannot be climbed many times during a human lifetime, is higher than all the others. Some breastfeeding mothers have experienced multiple orgasms followed by a tendency to fall asleep. One of them explained that when her baby was at the breast she could easily minimize or forget the little worries of daily life, on the condition that she had complete privacy, without any risk of being distracted. The words 'peace' and 'contentment' are commonly used when women try to describe their subjective experiences. It seems that there is infinity of degrees in the alterations of states of consciousness during the milk ejection reflex: from subtle almost imperceptible mood changes up to real orgasmic states.

Scientific interpretation of the 'milky way'

Through anatomical and physiological perspectives it is easy to interpret the 'milky way', to reach ecstatic states or at least to experience sensual pleasure. The breasts, particularly the nipples and the areolas, are perfectly equipped to be highly erogenous zones. They contain formations such as the 'genital corpuscles', which are end bulbs with a mulberry-like appearance found also in the clitoris and penis. They also contain the 'Golgi-Mazzoni tactile corpuscules' and the 'Vater-Pacini bodies', which consist of concentric layers or lamellae of connective tissue around a nerve ending and which are sensitive to deep or heavy pressure. All breast and nipple sensory activities finally converge on the neurons of the paraventricular nucleus of the hypothalamus (PVN), which is the common pathway for oxytocin secretion.

From a hormonal perspective, the similarities between the fetus ejection reflex, the sperm ejection reflex, the female genital orgasm and the milk ejection reflex are obvious. The same 'orgasmogenic cocktail' is involved in all episodes of sexual life. This cocktail always includes the release of oxytocin, the hormone of calmness and love, and the release of natural morphine, followed by a release of prolactin.

The important role of oxytocin in the milk ejection reflex has been understood and has been studied in depth in veterinary medicine since the middle of the twentieth century.[4] Interest in this reflex among humans has developed more recently. From human studies we have learned in particular that oxytocin release almost always starts before suckling. In a study involving ten breastfeeding mothers (five of them in early lactation and five of them in established lactation) it appeared that blood oxytocin concentrations increased three to ten minutes before suckling began.[5] In five women this occurred in response to the baby crying, in three it coincided with the baby becoming restless in expectation of the feed, while in two it corresponded with the mother preparing for the feed. These results clearly indicate that the release of oxytocin occurs in most women before the tactile stimulus of suckling. A second release of oxytocin follows in response to the suckling stimulus itself. We also learned from human studies that oxytocin must be released in a pulsatile manner to be effective. A Swedish study compared two groups of mothers and considered their hormonal response two days after birth when the baby was at the breast.[6] Twenty of them had given birth vaginally without any drugs, while seventeen had had an emergency cesarean. It appeared that the mothers who gave birth vaginally had significantly more pulses than those who had a cesarean. Furthermore, there was a correlation between the numbers of pulses two days after birth and the duration of exclusive breastfeeding. This study clearly demonstrates the strong links between the working of the oxytocin system during the birth process and lactation.

Increased maternal levels of natural opiates during lactation are also well established among non-human mammals and women.[7,8] Their roles as releasers of prolactin are well-documented. Endorphins are necessary components of the 'orgasmogenic cocktail'. After mentioning their importance during the birth process, during orgasms of genital sexuality and during lactation, we must also mention that the orgasm-like effects of opiates were perfectly described by the eighteenth century English physician John Jones. After studying the effects of ingestion of Tinct Opium ('Laudanum') he concluded: 'It has been compared not without good cause to a permanent gentle Degree of that Pleasure which Modesty forbids the name of.'[9] Since that time the possible orgasm-like effects of opiates have been confirmed, particularly after intravenous morphine injections.

Can the baby be ecstatic, even orgasmic?

While mothers can refer, in retrospect, to their subjective experiences when breastfeeding, it is more difficult to investigate the effects of morphine-like substances on the baby. Some babies seem to be on a high after being at the breast. The quivering of the lips and tongue followed by relaxation of the face into sleep have even been interpreted as the equivalent of oral orgasms. Such interpretations are plausible, since endorphins have been found in human milk, particularly during the first days following birth. Italian researchers found significant amounts of beta-endorphins in breast milk on the fourth day – if the baby had been born 'normally' by the vaginal route.[10,11] Human milk also contains substances similar to benzodiazepines (the well-known drugs Diazepam or Valium belong to this group).[12] The main effects of such substances are to relieve anxiety. We might therefore conclude that, when at the breast, the baby absorbs a sort of 'orgasmogenic cocktail'. The Swedish researchers who demonstrated benzodiazepine-like agents in milk hypothesized that such cocktails might be a phylogenetic relic of a time when our ancestors were constantly threatened by predators and when the baby had to keep quiet for survival.[13]

How cultural milieus interfere with the 'milky way'

Colostrum can be regarded as a symbol of the repression of instinctive forces, since babies in many cultures are usually deprived of it. The quasi-universal belief that colostrum is tainted or harmful is one of the countless ways in which cultures meddle with the newborn baby's relationship with his or her mother.[14] We can claim that delaying the initiation of breastfeeding has been the rule in almost all societies we know about. Western Europe is not a stranger to this universal rule. In Tudor and Stuart England, colostrum was openly regarded as a harmful substance, to be discarded.[15] The mother was not considered 'clean' after childbirth until the bloody discharge called 'lochia' had stopped flowing. She was not permitted to give the breast until after a religious service of purification and thanksgiving called 'churching'. Meanwhile the baby was given a purgative made from such things as butter, honey and sugar, oil of sweet almonds or sugared wine. Paintings from that time show the newborn infant fed with a spoon while the mother recovered in bed. In Brittany the baby was not put to the breast before baptism, which took place at the age of two or three days. The Bretons of old believed that if the baby swallowed milk before the ceremony, the devil might enter the baby's body along with the milk.

The duration of breastfeeding is undoubtedly influenced by family structures. Since human societies organize mating and create marriage rules, they also indirectly influence the duration of breastfeeding. Nobody knows exactly what the physiological ideal for the duration of breastfeeding is among humans. For any other mammal, the answer is simple – almost as simple as for the duration of pregnancy. For example, after spending 230 days in the womb, the baby chimpanzee is fed by its mother for two years; a bottle-nosed dolphin is breastfed for 16 months. For human beings the answer is much more imprecise, although a physiological ideal can be deduced as a reference point. Comparing human beings with other mammals and taking into account the duration of our life in the womb, our degree of maturity at birth, our lifespan, the special nutritional needs of our big brain, tooth development, and so forth, we might conclude that breastfeeding among humans was originally maintained for a matter of years rather than a few months.

As a matter of fact it appears that before the advent of lifelong strict monogamy as the only morally acceptable kind of marriage, most human babies were breastfed for two to four years. Of course we must take into account that there has always been great diversity amongst polygamic societies. Because of the usual statistical distribution of men and women it makes sense that polygyny (where one husband has several wives) has been by far more frequent than polyandry (where one wife has several husbands). (The rare polyandric societies that have existed, such as among the Toda in India, or in Tibet, were characterized by an excess of men). Significantly, in most polygynic societies sexual intercourse was forbidden during the lactation period. We should also note that this rule was probably not too hard to respect since prolactin is an inhibitor of libido and since non-human mammals are therefore not receptive to males during lactation.

The advent of strict monogamy is recent in the history of mankind. It is mostly a Greek-Roman phenomenon. The Old Testament gives us an idea of when cultural changes occurred because in the earliest texts there are many examples of respectable polygamous patriarchies – for example Abraham, Jacob, David, and Solomon – but similar examples cannot be found in the more recent biblical texts, particularly in the New Testament.

As soon as monogamy was considered the norm, difficulties in breastfeeding, even obstacles, appeared. In Greek society there were slaves called *titthai,* whose role was to breastfeed the children of their masters for six months. Women of high society were afraid of jeopardizing their health and their silhouette and also of neglecting their 'duties' by breastfeeding themselves. In the most recent texts of the Old Testament, Jeremiah also referred to an aversion to breastfeeding. He was talking to those who wanted to be fashionable, who therefore refused to breastfeed, when he commented: 'Even the sea monsters offer their breast to their offspring.' It was for the same reasons that until recently women had recourse to wet nurses in Western Europe over the last two hundred years. City women who were rich enough used to send their babies to wet nurses living in the country. These wet nurses belonged to a low socio-economic class and some of them were also prostitutes. It is worth noting here that both wet nurses and prostitutes in monogamous societies can be seen as mercenaries who supply substitutes for love, either maternal or marital. It is also important to note that as a result of these wet nurse practices, for many centuries a great part of the female population had no exposure to the love hormones associated with breastfeeding and the milk ejection reflex.

The practice of using wet nurses continued until the nineteenth century, in spite of eloquent, powerful and authoritative comments against the practice. For example, the Jewish Talmud encourages mothers to nurse until eighteen months to two years; two years of nursing is recommended in the Koran and – historically – Julius Caesar had regretted that babies of Patricians were not being given mothers' milk. Jean-Jacques Rousseau, on the other hand, made breastfeeding fashionable among elegant Parisians and women in the European upper classes in the eighteenth century, by associating it with a return to nature[16]. 'The fashionable mamma', an etching of James Gillray English dated 1796 (displayed in the British Museum), suggests that Rousseau's theories had a strong impact on breastfeeding practices at the time.

Infant feeding with non-human milk is another result of the attitude that led to the *titthai*, the wet nurse, and also the nursing slave in some American states. In some parts of the world – such as in Iceland – the use of cow's milk became the norm. Icelandic babies were not breastfed at all during the seventeenth and the eighteenth centuries[17] but were given cow's milk, cream, and chewed fish. At that time infant mortality rates were the highest in Europe, in the region of 300 per thousand and many women had more than ten children.[18] A change in religious imagery probably played a role in terms of encouraging women to abandon breastfeeding since at that time the influence of institutionalized religion was enormous: after the Reformation, the Virgin Mary lost her supremely important position in popular religious practice and the paintings of Jesus at the breast disappeared. Dr Guojon Guonason, a retired obstetrician from Reykjavik who has studied the history of infant feeding in his country, deduced that in 1849 while there were no authorized midwives, only eight medical doctors and no hospital, there were 249 churches.

* * *

When medical institutions take control

The particular case of Iceland strongly suggests that before the twentieth century it was largely religious institutions that influenced cultural milieus and many aspects of people's lifestyles, involving practices such as infant feeding. In the twentieth century, by contrast, there has been a marked decrease in the influence of the Church and medical institutions have had a far great influence on all aspects of our reproductive and sexual lives. Doctors have found medical reasons for interfering with the relationship between mothers and newborn babies. However, it must be said that such new medical rituals had no spectacular effect on the initiation of breastfeeding, since in any case until the 1970s nobody was aware that breastfeeding could start in the hour following birth when the physiological processes of labor and birth are not disturbed. Through the development of hospital births, the tradition of separating babies from their mothers and denying them breast milk was continued, since most newborn babies spent their first days following birth in nurseries. These babies were fed – either mother's milk, or artificial milk, or both – according to strict rules and pre-established schedules. As a result, for several decades it was the medical institutions that dictated infant feeding patterns.

A great diversity of new factors influencing infant feeding patterns appeared during the post Second World War baby boom. The fast development of the food industry had an obvious and spectacular effect on breastfeeding rates. Such concepts as 'humanized milk' subliminally implied that differences between human milk and artificial milk might be eliminated. This partly explains the spectacular decrease in rates of breastfeeding in the 1950s and 1960s in developed countries and soon after in developing countries. At the same time, the dominant form of feminism devalued activities that are specifically female (giving birth, breastfeeding, mothering, etc.), while another form of feminism, on the contrary, challenged the messages disseminated by the medical institution and the food industry. A new generation of women's groups appeared, which included, for example, one group of seven mothers from Illinois who focused on breastfeeding. These women felt that services provided by experts were extremely limited and inadequate and, as a result, they created La Leche League in 1956. This was initially a mother-to-mother help group, which eventually became a huge international organization, and which is still in existence and thriving.

Institutionalized medicine could not ignore a great diversity of new challenges. Attitudes that had previously been dominant were gradually reconsidered and new concepts appeared in most industrialized countries. 'Rooming-in' is one of them and involves placing the newborn baby in a crib beside the mother's bed so that the mother herself can care for her baby while she is in hospital. This practice is undoubtedly one way of facilitating the initiation of breastfeeding, although at the very time when more and more health professionals started to realize the negative side effects of conventional medical practices and were trying to facilitate the mother-infant relationship and the initiation of breastfeeding, the evolution of obstetrics led to new ways to interfere.

The increased safety of the cesarean and the increased use of pharmacological substitutes for maternal hormones – in particular epidural anesthesia, drips of synthetic oxytocin and drugs for placental delivery – both created entirely new scenarios. For the first time in the history of mankind, most women could have babies without using their own hormones. When the strong connections between birth physiology and lactation physiology are considered, the current unsatisfactory breastfeeding statistics in places where women cannot give birth are not at all surprising.

Today the promotion of breastfeeding is one of the priorities of most public health organizations. In many countries, such as Brazil and China (countries with skyrocketing cesarean rates), campaigns are to a large extent in the hands of governmental departments. The public health way of promoting breastfeeding can be seen as effective inasmuch as most people in our societies now believe that 'Breast is Best'. (This is a conclusion I have drawn as a result of my own unofficial survey of taxi drivers in different countries.) However, this shift in attitude has not significantly affected breastfeeding statistics, which must lead us to question how useful these modern direct methods of promotion are. There is an enormous gap between knowledge, awareness and intentions on the one hand, and statistical data on the other. In many countries the duration of breastfeeding falls far short of that recommended by national plans. Our priority now, therefore, should not be to promote breastfeeding; it should be to understand why in our societies lactation is difficult and cannot continue as long as intended. In order to find an answer, we need to address a very basic, but necessary and paradoxically new question: 'How does the capacity to breastfeed develop?'

The need to conceptualize new questions regarding the capacity to breastfeed is better understood if we relate the capacity to breastfeed to the capacity to love. The value of love and the value of breastfeeding are well accepted but, in both cases, the behaviors are not obviously influenced by shared awareness. Love has been promoted since time immemorial. Spiritual heroes, religious leaders, philosophers, poets, moralists and philanthropists of all kinds have used a great diversity of terms to encourage the expression of love's many facets. Since the word 'love' has a positive connotation in most languages, it might be that its promotion has been effective. But, when considering the behavior of twenty-first century humans, we don't need long arguments to call into question the usefulness of the campaign to promote love. This is why this analogy between breastfeeding and the capacity to love has inspired the provocative title of one of the newsletters from the Primal Health Research Centre: 'Is promoting breastfeeding as useless as the promotion of love?'[19]

7

THE UNEQUALLY EQUIPPED SEXES

Our overview, from a physiological perspective, of all ecstatic states human beings can experience during their reproductive and sexual lives could lead us to identify an 'orgasmogenic cocktail'. This is roughly the same irrespective of gender or episode in a person's sexual life. However, as students of human nature, we cannot improve our understanding of male-female relationships without changing our focus and also looking at differences. Some of these differences are obvious inasmuch as men appear to be able to use only one ladder, the genital ladder, while women have at their disposal the 'birth ladder' and the 'milky way', in addition to any genital ladder they might climb.

From physiology to mythology and proverbs

Even within the framework of genital sexuality there are gender differences. In her pioneering study of oxytocin levels during sexual arousal and orgasm Marie Carmichael noticed that levels of oxytocin during self-stimulation before orgasm were higher among women than among men.[1] She also observed that levels were higher among women than men during any one orgasm, and that multi-orgasmic women reached a higher peak in oxytocin levels during a second orgasm. In another study Carmichael's team found that in the case of multi-orgasmic women any increase in oxytocin level correlated with subjective reports of orgasmic intensity.[2] In the light of this new generation of research, also taking into account the refractory phase after any male ejaculatory orgasm, we conclude that women are physiologically better equipped than men to reach high intensity genital orgasms.

The scientific study of the different facets of love provides answers to questions that were repressed during the long orgasmophobic phase of human history. Until recently mortal human beings did not dare to wonder if women could enjoy more or less pleasure than men during sexual intercourse. However the question has been addressed by myths involving gods, such as the myth of Tiresias. Once Tiresias saw two snakes mating; since they felt disturbed they attacked him. During the fight the female was killed. This is how Tiresias turned into a woman. Seven years later, when Tiresias was still a woman, the episode of the snakes reoccured. This time the male was killed and Tiresias was turned back into a man. Then, when Zeus and his wife Hera had a disagreement about which sex enjoys the most pleasure during intercourse they decided to let Tiresias judge, since he had experienced both forms of sexual pleasure. Tiresias said that if sexual pleasure could be put on a scale from one to ten, men were at one and women at three times three. There are striking similarities between the myth of Tiresias and an Indian proverb around 500 AD:

'The woman's impetuosity on love and her delight in love's pleasure are eight times as great as the man's'.[3]

When modern physiology, mythology, and old Indian proverbs are in agreement we might conclude that another step has been made in terms of understanding the laws of nature.

The intimate links between oxytocin and female hormones

The strong connections between oxytocin and the female hormones called estrogens represent an unavoidable physiological basis for interpreting gender differences. We must bear in mind that until the late 1970s estrogens were considered the main hormonal agents involved in maternal love. A strong interest for the hormonal aspect of maternal behavior had developed after the historical experiment by Terkel and Rosenblatt, who injected virgin rats with blood taken from mother rats within 48 hours of their giving birth.[4] The virgin rats behaved like mothers. Terkel and Rosenblatt had demonstrated that, immediately after birth, there are hormones that influence maternal behavior in the blood of mother rats. This is why, in the 1970s, Rosenblatt and Siegel, in the USA, who were studying rats,[5] and Poindron and Le Neindre in France, who were studying sheep,[6] looked in particular at the effects of estrogens. Furthermore, it had been noticed that female rats that are about to give birth (a situation associated with high levels of estrogens) immediately respond maternally towards newborns, while it is only after prolonged physical proximity to newborns and habituation to pup stimuli that virgin rats begin to exhibit all components of maternal behavior.[7] We can easily understand why, until recently, there was a prevailing view that the high estrogens levels and the rapid decline in progesterone levels occurring in the period surrounding birth were the hormonal events activating the maternal behavior.

We can also understand why, until recently, there was a widespread lack of interest in the possible behavioral effects of oxytocin. Researchers (and practitioners) knew that intravenous infusions failed to influence maternal behavior.[8] Furthermore, lesions of the posterior pituitary gland which prevented the release of oxytocin into the blood stream did not block maternal behavior.[9] These negative results were interpreted as conclusive evidence that oxytocin played no role in maternal behavior and these beliefs remained almost unchallenged as long the prevailing view persisted that oxytocin was solely a peripheral hormone released into the bloodstream by the posterior pituitary gland.

However an interest in the behavioral effects of oxytocin – which had remained intact among only a small number of scientists inspired by Niles Newton – was rekindled in the late 1970s by new anatomical evidence, which suggested that oxytocin might be released directly into the brain. This new anatomical data inspired the historical experiment by Cort Pedersen and Arthur Prange, presented for the first time at the National Academy of Sciences, USA, in December 1979. Pedersen and Prange injected oxytocin directly into the cerebral ventricles of intact virgin rats[10] and found that half the animals developed the full spectrum of maternal behavior in less than an hour after treatment. (At this point, it is worth remembering that there have been so many studies of maternal behavior among rats that its main components are well-known: nest building, retrieval and grouping of pups within the nest, licking and cleaning of pups, and crouching over pups in a nurturing posture.) In this new experiment the rats that responded to oxytocin with maternal behavior were in stages of estrous cycle associated with rising, elevated, or recently elevated estrogens. Not only did this mean that Pedersen and Prange were demonstrating that oxytocin has behavioral effects, they were also suggesting that the behavioral effects of oxytocin are estrogen dependent.

A Japanese team tested this hypothesis. By studying the effects of estrogen treatment on blood oxytocin levels of ovariectomized rats they confirmed that estrogens affect both the release of and the response to oxytocin.[11]

Since these pioneering studies, the nature of the connections between oxytocin and estrogens has been clarified. Estrogens have been found to act on two different receptors, the alpha and the beta types. We understand today that it is via the beta-receptors that estrogens modulate the oxytocin system.[12,13,14] Our current understanding of the oxytocin-estrogens connection offers an easy interpretation of the frequent waning of women's libido with age, when the levels of estrogens are decreasing.

The intimate link between vasopressin and male hormones

Vasopressin and oxytocin are 'sister hormones'. They are closely related in chemical composition. Both of them are made of nine amino acids. Both of them have been present in the chain of animal evolution for millions of years. Both of them are produced among males and females in the supraoptic and paraventricular nuclei of the hypothalamus. Both of them function in two parallel ways, as hormones in the blood stream released by the posterior pituitary and as signaling substances in the central nervous system. Both of them have strong connections with sexual hormones.

One of the main differences between these 'sister hormones' is that while estrogens act as oxytocin enhancers, it is with the male hormone testosterone that vasopressin has strong links.[15,16] In other words, while oxytocin is the main component of what Kerstin Uvnäs-Moberg calls the 'calm and connection system', vasopressin is more closely related to the 'flight and fight system'.[17] Vasopressin can initiate aggressive behaviors, particularly aggressiveness of males towards other males. One of the specific effects of vasopressin is to decrease urine production and to facilitate the retention of salt and fluid; at the same time it contracts blood vessels and tends to increase blood pressure. Mammals need to conserve fluids if the situation appears dangerous and if there is a risk of wounds that would cause blood loss. These are situations associated with the release of hormones of the adrenaline family and it is probable that during a male orgasm the fight and flight system can more or less modify the typical orgasmogenic cocktail. It is significant that sexual activity can involve some sort of violence, particularly male violence. There have been reports of men beating their partners, or shivering, or having goose bumps during an orgasm. It is as if the basic orgasmogenic cocktail is to a certain extent more easily altered among men. This is another way of concluding that men and women are not a priori equally equipped in terms of orgasmic capabilities.

8

THE HIGHWAYS TO TRANSCENDENCE

In the current scientific context, orgasmic states are becoming necessary objects of scrutiny to improve our understanding of the human phenomenon. Of course all mammals activate their reward systems during the different episodes of their reproductive life. Of course among all mammals there are fetus ejection reflexes, sperm ejection reflexes, and milk ejection reflexes. Of course the subjective aspect of these ejection reflexes will always remain mysterious in other species than ours, since only human beings are capable of speech – so we can assume that the coital consciousness of a chimpanzee will always remain inexpressible! However, in spite of such difficulties, we can echo Desmond Morris, who called *Homo sapiens* 'the sexiest primate alive'. The sophisticated brain cataclysms at the top of the birth ladder and the genital ladder are specifically human. There is an undisputable reason for this: the development of the brain – our main sexual organ – has reached an unprecedented order of magnitude in our species only. Whatever a person's perspective when studying human nature, it is necessary to take into account *Homo sapiens'* status as a mammal with a gigantic brain of enormous complexity.

Escaping from space and time reality

It is now clear that all ecstatic states related to our sexual life involve intense activity of the archaic primitive brain structures inseparable from our basic adaptive systems, while the new brain (the neocortex) is put at rest. Since the neocortex gives us access to space-bound, time-bound reality, we can interpret subjective orgasmic experiences as opportunities to escape from space and time-bound reality. It is noticeable that orgasmic states have rarely been considered in the context of changed levels of consciousness. Since the 'scientification of love' is bound to include the scientification of orgasmic states, one cannot avoid questions about the functions of such changes of consciousness. Today it is well accepted that when fighting is impossible there is only one way to protect our health in adverse circumstances, and that is to escape. There are many ways to escape and to refuse to submit to a situation – going into another reality than space and time reality is just one of them.

This new vision of the functions of orgasmic and ecstatic states is reminiscent of the most important advances in our understanding of health and disease over the past few decades. This has been the identification of the prototype of pathogenic (disease creating) situations, which entails being trapped in adverse or threatening circumstances and being unable to either fight or flee. When we can only passively submit, our health tends to deteriorate.[1] On the other hand, being in a position to take the initiative is health enhancing.

The story began with simple experiments with rats, cats and dogs that became sick after receiving a series of electric shocks.[2, 3] It was not the electric shocks themselves that made the animals ill, but the submissive state they were in at the time of receiving the shocks. Their health was not endangered when they had the opportunity to fight a companion (another animal in the cage) or if they had some means of escape, even though all the groups studied finally received the same number of electric shocks. There is an altered hormonal balance during 'uncontrollable adverse events' which suggests that when we have lost all hope and given up, a self-destructive process starts. Much of the data published in the medical literature confirms that the results of such experiments with non-human mammals can be transposed to human subjects. Among humans several situations of 'learned helplessness', 'learned hopelessness', and 'inhibition of action' have been widely explored.

All mammals, including human beings, experience a great diversity of situations in which they feel trapped, and therefore have many occasional reasons to try to escape. However, as far as the need to escape is concerned, human beings are special. Once more it is the power of our neo-cortical supercomputer that makes us different from other mammals. Because our new brain supports the concepts of time, space and boundaries, including the limits of our lifespan, and because we speak, we know that we'll die. This is a reality we need to escape from now and then. Reaching the tops of the genital ladder, the birth ladder, or the milky way are human physiological means of escaping now and then from space- and time-bound reality.

Transcendent emotional states

By presenting orgasmic states as opportunities to escape from space and time reality, we suggest that human beings might have access to an out-of-time-and-space reality. In other words orgasmic states might be looked at in terms of transcendent emotional states. An infinite range of transcendent emotions in terms of purity and intensity have been reported, from the discreet 'oceanic feeling' we might experience on a beach at sunset to the pure and intense 'peak experience'. Since the 'peak experience' has been reported in a great number of cultures, there are many other ways of describing it – 'cosmic experience', 'mystical union', 'enlightenment', 'nirvana', 'mystical ecstasy', and so on.

In order to justify the inclusion of orgasmic states within this new framework it is necessary to consider an overview of the many previous descriptions that have been made of transcendent emotional states. It is well accepted that transcendent emotions are more likely to occur in certain situations, such as darkness, solitude, silence... Artistic activities – those artifices employed by humans to harmonize their two brains – can induce transcendent emotions. In any artistic activity a technique – made possible by the specifically human neocortex – is serving a function that, in turn, is controlled by the older structures. The technique of a musician makes it possible to transmit emotions through sound. The technique of a painter can transmit emotions through visual signals. Poetry is another way of expressing emotions by means of one elaborated form of communication called 'language'. The technique of a dancer tends to arouse emotions induced by body movements and rhythms. Gastronomy is related to digestive functions; the art of the perfumer to our sense of smell; eroticism to the mating instinct. There is no physiological function that cannot be the basis of some artistic activity, and all forms of artistic activity have the power to induce subtle or intense emotions that can be experienced as transcendent. Singing, by definition, offers a particularly apt way of harmonizing the two brains, since melody and rhythm are associated with the use of words to communicate emotions. Furthermore, certain works of art – Gothic cathedrals, Indian temples, the Egyptian Sphinx, Sanskrit hymns, Bach music, Gregorian plainsong, for example – all came into being originally because of man's need to convey transcendent emotions.

Artistic activities are not the only ways human beings have used to catch a glimpse of realities that go beyond time and space. There are many roads leading to transcendence. Similar roads have been widely used in a great diversity of cultural milieus. This is the case with shamanism, hypnotic trance, prayer, meditation, fasting, and psychedelic drugs, for example.

Certain pathological conditions, particularly epileptic seizures, have also been presented as possible roads to transcendence.[4] It has been pointed out, for example, that during his conversion on the road to Damascus, Saint Paul had three days of blindness, fell down to the ground, and experienced ecstatic visions. Muhammad described falling episodes accompanied by visual and auditory hallucinations. Joseph Smith, who founded Mormonism, reported lapses of consciousness and speech arrest, and once found himself lying on the ground. As for Joan of Arc, a great light accompanied the voice she heard.

It seems that, in general, extreme transcendent emotions – peak experiences – cannot be induced on purpose. They just occur unexpectedly. The classical analyses of peak experiences by researchers such as Richard Buke[5] and Arthur Deikman[6] suggest striking similarities with subjective descriptions of intense orgasmic states. A peak experience is described as a paroxysm, a climax, a culmination, and there is invariably a speedy return to 'normality'. The 'peak experience' is characterized by a consciousness of the Oneness of everything – 'All in One and One in All' – and also, by the sense of timelessness, which implies a sense of immortality. 'Peak experiences' are associated with feelings of surrender and a sense of infinite wellbeing. A peak experience can be followed by a real transformation of the person. Interestingly, most women who gave birth through an authentic fetus ejection reflex and who were in an ecstatic state at the time of the very first contact with the newborn baby claim that they have been transformed by the experience.

Hard-wired emotional states

Any in depth exploration of human nature is bound to address the issue of transcendent mysteries. Transcendent emotional states that provide access to an out-of-space-and-time reality are universal. They are at the root of all religions. It is mostly through religious institutions that cultural milieus channel and control the expression of the need for transcendence. All societies develop, promote, and give directions to paths towards transcendence that are culturally acceptable. For example prayer, religious music and shamanic trances are organized by religions to a greater or lesser degree; they are also regulated according to pre-established schedules.

In the age of monotheist religions, there is a tendency to turn a blind eye to the hard-wired transcendent emotional states as the root of all religions. Rationalistic thinkers are not interested in what Albert Einstein called 'cosmic religious feeling', which others have termed an 'oceanic feeling'. Rationalistic thinkers are those who are unable to take into consideration realities other than the reality to which they have access via their neocortical supercomputer. They mainly discuss the existence of God, without realizing that the concept of one unique God as a paternal figure was created too recently in the history of mankind to be considered the origin of all religions. For example Friedrich Nietzsche made his famous proclamation that God is dead. In his mind the death of God was also the end of religions. For Sigmund Freud, the belief in God is related to an absolute state of dependency in infancy and the need to be protected by one's father. His interpretations are not valid outside patriarchal societies regulated by monotheist religions. Similar comments might be made about Karl Marx, who proclaimed that in 'the country of reason' the existence of God cannot have any meaning, about Bertrand Russell, who participated with Father Frederick Copleston in the famous BBC 'debate on the existence of God', or about Richard Dawkins, the author of *The God Delusion*. Questions about 'life after death' also translate the widespread tendency to ignore the emotional states at the root of all religions: the word 'after' includes the concept of time, while transcendence is about out-of-time reality.

In the current scientific climate any study of orgasmic/ecstatic states related to our reproductive life should lead us to conclude that access to transcendence implies first a reduced activity of the neocortex. This is a new way to present transcendence as an aspect of the human phenomenon. Because the prerequisite for access to transcendence has not been well understood until now, the ambition of many scientists has been to locate the seat of spirituality instead of focusing on the specifically human obstacles. As is well known, Descartes, in *Les Passions de l'Ame*, chose the pineal gland as the seat of the soul because it appeared to him to be the only organ in the brain that was not bilaterally duplicated and because he believed, erroneously, that it was uniquely human. Since Descartes countless physiologists, psychologists, philosophers and religionists, inspired by the central location of this gland in the brain, have been speculating about the pineal's function in relation to the spirit and the soul. Interestingly, too, brain mapping carried out during a traditional Chinese religious meditation called 'Quiet Sitting' has showed an activation of the pineal gland.[7,8] The media was keen to comment on these findings, as if the seat of spirituality had been discovered, or at least confirmed. Our interpretation is that an increased activity of the pineal gland suggests a release of melatonin, and the well-known effect of melatonin is to reduce the activity of the neocortex.

While, until recently, the ambition of scientists was often to locate the seat of spirituality, some twenty-first century academics have been granted millions of dollars in order to investigate whether religious beliefs are hard-wired or the effects of cultural conditioning. Do we really need a budget of millions of dollars to realize that transcendent emotional states occur when the activity of the neocortex is at rest, therefore when cultural conditioning has been largely eliminated?

The time has come to try to interpret our current difficulties in recognizing the universal need for transcendence as the real origin of all religions. One of the reasons for these difficulties might be that for thousands of years all cultures have controlled, channeled, replaced, and finally suppressed the physiological highways to transcendence. These highways are strongly related to the urge to transmit our genes and to survive as a species. The need to survive is not imprinted in the neocortex. It is hard-wired. It is outside the field of rationality.

9

BONOBOS, DOLPHINS AND HUMANS

When studying human orgasms in the framework of brain physiology and changes in levels of consciousness, we could echo Desmond Morris and present the 'big-brained ape' as 'the sexiest primate alive'. The sudden and dramatic changes in the comparative activity of the different parts of our gigantic and sophisticated brain during orgasms may be considered specifically human.

Challenging common beliefs

Despite this, we must challenge the widespread pre-conceived idea that human beings are also special since they have – to a certain extent – dissociated sexuality and reproduction. There is a general rule among mammals that the female is sexually attractive and receptive to the male only during a few days of her cycle. Because human beings have sexual intercourse at any phase of the cycle and after the age of reproduction, they are usually presented as unique exceptions to the rule. In other words it has often been considered specifically human to have sex just for pleasure. We must also challenge the idea that face-to-face copulation is uniquely human, even a sort of cultural innovation that needs to be taught to preliterate people – hence the term 'missionary position'. The apparent human exceptions lead us to explore the links between our species and a small number of non-human mammals, particularly dolphins and bonobos.

Dolphins are known to have sex very frequently, in many different ways, for reasons other than reproduction, and they sometimes engage in acts of a homosexual nature. Copulation takes place face-to-face and though many species of dolphins engage in lengthy foreplay, the actual act is usually only brief, but may be repeated several times within a short time span. Various dolphin species have even been known to engage in sexual behavior with other dolphin species. Occasionally, dolphins will also show sexual behavior towards other animals, including humans. Bonobos (otherwise known as pygmy chimpanzees, or *Pan paniscus*), like us, belong to the chimpanzee family. They live in the swampy equatorial forests of the left bank of the Congo River. Their sexual life has been studied in particular by Frans de Waal at the San Diego zoo[1] and it seems they are an oversexed species. They often copulate face-to-face and the frontal orientation of the bonobo vulva and clitoris both strongly suggest that the female genitalia are adapted for this position. During sexual intercourse the females have been heard emitting grunts and squeals that probably reflect orgasmic experiences, which perhaps explains why sex, among bonobos, is not just for reproduction – it is the key to their social life. Bonobos become sexually aroused remarkably easily, and they express this excitement in a variety of mounting positions and forms of genital contact. Perhaps the bonobo's most typical sexual pattern is genito-genital rubbing between adult females. The two females rub their genital swellings laterally together. Male bonobos, too, may engage in pseudocopulation; they often perform a back to back variation, one male briefly rubbing his scrotum against the buttocks of another. These mammals also practice so-called penis fencing, in which two males hang face-to-face from a branch, rubbing their erect penises together.

A new vision of human nature

The fact that other mammals also separate sex and reproduction and also copulate face-to-face suggests the need to consider unexplored similarities or links between these species and ourselves. One possible link is a special relationship with an aquatic environment. That dolphins have a special relationship with water is obvious, but it is also quite obvious for the bonobos, who live in swamps and love swimming; this is in marked contrast to common chimpanzees, who hate water and panic in it. As for humans, some explanations are needed because, for many thousands of years, countless philosophers and scholars who pronounced on human nature did so without noticing that *Homo sapiens* has similarities to aquatic mammals.

I became aware of the power of water on humans in a surprising way and in an unexpected environment. In a French state hospital, where I was in charge of the surgical unit, I practiced all kinds of emergency surgery, including cesareans. As I was an overworked surgeon, I wondered whether it might be possible to make labor easier. It soon became apparent that many women wanted to take a shower or bath during labor and I soon became particularly interested in the incredible attraction to water some women experienced while in labor. Our medical team therefore responded to what seemed to constitute a real need.[2] First of all, as a temporary measure, we had a big inflatable garden paddling pool installed, which could be filled with warm water. Later on we installed a very large, round, deep-blue bath, which we had plumbed in. I had a revelation the day a woman gave birth on the floor before the pool was actually full. All she needed, to release her inhibitions, was to see the blue water and to hear the noise of water filling the pool. I was able to see the importance of water as a symbol and the role it can play in human sexuality. I was able to establish an analogy between the power of water during labor and the well-known erotic power of water.[3]

Today there are new ways of interpreting the magic power that water appears to have on human beings. The theory that humans must have evolved in a coastal ecosystem, along lakes, estuaries and oceans, is becoming widely accepted. This makes sense because the coastal food chain is the only one which can provide all the essential nutrients needed to develop a gigantic brain: very long chain polyunsaturated fatty acids of the Omega-3 family, iodine and a good balance in other brain selective minerals such as iron, copper, zinc, magnesium and selenium are all present. After all, it is difficult to believe that, after leaving the trees, our clever and curious ancestors did not discover the richness of the coastal food chain, bearing in mind that the bones of the famous Lucy were found among turtle and crocodile eggs, and crab claws. Furthermore we have evidence to suggest that during a recent phase in the evolution of our species, about 164,000 years ago, our ancestors included in their diet sources of marine life, particularly shellfish. This is the conclusion of studies conducted at Pinnacle Point, on the south coast of South Africa.[4]

Apart from brain size there are dozens of other features which make us different from our very close relative, the common chimpanzee: nakedness, a layer of fat attached to the skin, a comparatively low basal body temperature, sweating for thermo-regulation, the development of a prominent nose, large empty sinuses on each side of the nasal cavities, a low larynx, a reduced number of red blood cells and anatomical particularities of hands and feet being among the main differences. All these features are suggestive of adaptation to a semi-aquatic environment.

We must also focus on one feature that makes humans different from other land mammals, particularly common chimpanzees. This is the general shape of our body, with the hind limbs forming an extension of the trunk, which makes us streamlined, like all sea mammals. This body shape makes us well adapted for gathering food in shallow water and therefore for walking and running on two feet. Human babies, for example, can stay erect and walk in water before being able to walk on dry land. Bonobos, who live in swamps, often walk upright even during ground locomotion and the general shape of their bodies is not very different from ours. This streamlined body shape, which is an important factor influencing sexual behavior, clearly makes face-to-face copulation easy and face-to-face copulation results in a greater amount of skin-to-skin contact between partners. Indeed, we may assume that this large amount of contact intensely activates physiological reward systems, which must lead to a tendency to repeat the experience of sexual contact as often as possible, even during infertile periods of the female reproductive cycle.

Today, all chapters of human anatomy, physiology, behavior, pathology, and evolutionary medicine must be rewritten in the light of this so-called 'aquatic ape theory'. This new vision of *Homo sapiens* was first proposed independently by Max Westenhofer in Berlin (1942) and by Alister Hardy in Oxford (1960), but it is the British science writer Elaine Morgan who has championed the cause in her book[5,6,7] and in the seminars she has organized in order to constantly update and strengthen the theory. It was in fact at her last seminar in San Rafael, California, in June 1994, that I associated the human pregnancy disease 'eclampsia' with evolutionary medicine for the very first time in a presentation.

I proposed that eclampsia is the price some human beings have to pay for having a large brain, while being more or less separated from the seafood chain.[8] I suggested that human eclampsia is the expression of a maternal fetal conflict in a species where the priority is to satisfy the specific nutritional needs of the developing brain. We learn from veterinary medicine that maternal fetal conflicts express differently according to the characteristics of the species. For example, among dogs, the priority is to feed the bones and the pregnancy disease is related to a lack of calcium, while in herbivorous mammals, where the priority is to satisfy the needs in carbohydrates, the pregnancy disease is mostly a hypoglycemia. We are currently testing this hypothesis through studies of nutrition in pregnancy that are inspired by huge geographical differences in the incidence of the disease. In a low-income population at risk of eclampsia, in the peripheral part of Rio de Janeiro, pregnant women are given food supplements (sardine sandwiches). The objective is to evaluate the effects of such supplements on the risks of this pregnancy disease. This is the first trial of the effects of food supplementation on the risks of eclampsia. The acronym FISH hypothesis (Fetal Interference in Sapiens Homo) is a reminder that, via the placenta, the fetus interferes with maternal physiology for its own benefit. Until now there have only been studies looking at the effects of micronutrients.[9]

It is thanks to the work of Michael Crawford as an expert in the specific nutritional needs of the brain that our new understanding of the emergence of Man has been dramatically reinforced and has reached a high degree of credibility.[10] More recently the point of view of Stephen Cunnane, another authoritative expert in brain nutritional needs, should convince anyone that the main environmental influence in human development was the adaptation to a 'shore-based' diet.[11]

The fantasy life of human beings also needs to be re-explored in the current scientific context. From the coast, our ancestors could face the immensity of the ocean. They could develop a sense of infinity. They could not ignore the 'oceanic feeling' as a basic transcendent emotional state. They could not ignore the 'other reality' they also had access to during orgasmic and ecstatic experiences.

THE EVOLUTIONARY ADVANTAGES
OF ORGASMOPHOBIA

Shame, guilt, and fear

Since the advent of the literate phase of the history of
mankind, many cultures and civilizations have disappeared.
A small number of them may be deemed 'successful', since
they have survived or have emerged as new cultural enti-
ties. In order to identify the laws that govern the evolution
of cultural milieus, the first step is to focus on the main features shared by 'successful' human groups. One of the
most intriguing of these features is the association of orgasmic states with shame, guilt and fear.

Our vocabulary indicates that this widespread 'orgasmophobia' is deep-rooted. For example 'pudenda' is used in
English as the scientific term for the external genital organs,
which are innerved by the 'pudendal' nerves and receive
their blood via the 'pudendal arteries' (in Spanish they
refer to nervios pudendos, and in Portuguese to nervo
pudendo) . The root of these terms is the Latin verb 'pud-
ere', which means 'to be ashamed'. In French the word

'pudeur' (sense of modesty) has a strong virtuous connotation, while 'nerfs honteux' and 'vaisseaux honteux' ('honteux' means shameful) are anatomical terms related to the genitalia. In German 'scham' (ie. shame) is the first components of many words related to the genitalia and the pubic region: 'Schamhaare' (pubic hair), 'Schamlippe' (labia majoris), 'Schamhaft' (genitalia), 'Schamberg' (mons pubis), 'Schamfuge'(pubic symphysis), etc. In Chinese the pubic bone is called 'chigu', which literally means 'shame-bone' It is also significant that in Japanese the penis is often called 'the son', suggesting that the use of a specific or too explicit term would be a violation of the norms of the culture that would induce a feeling of shame.

Holy scriptures, myths and legends also translate and transmit the widespread orgasmophobia. For example, in our culture, conceiving a baby without sin is considered a miracle. There are still today women who are ashamed to be pregnant: it is as if they feel obliged to confess sinful experiences. There are also women who feel ashamed when reaching an ecstatic state during the milk ejection reflex.

We can conclude that the foundations of our orgasmophobic cultural milieus include the concept of shame. It is therefore essential to analyze and clarify the meaning of this term. 'Shame' (like 'scham' in German) has an Indo-European root, *isikam*, meaning 'to hide'. It is an emotional state associated with the need to avert the eyes, to hang the head, to hide or cover up. The expression of shame is undoubtedly hard-wired. Infants can lower their heads and avert their gaze when a parent scolds them. While guilt is just a warning sign that we have done something wrong, shame is a powerful emotional state that implies a loss of self-esteem and even a disgust with oneself. Shame, as a dreaded situation, has a social function. It is directed towards small groups or individuals who violate the cultural rules. By keeping people in line, it plays an important role in maintaining the cohesion of human groups. Orgasmophobia – the fear of orgasmic states – is basically the phobia of shameful situations.

We have underlined that women and men are not equally equipped regarding their orgasmic function. We can wonder if they are equal regarding shame as a well-defined emotional state. It is an inescapable question, since in our culture women have borne the original sexual shame, and since virginity has been for ages considered the purest and holiest state for women. Freud, who coined the word 'hysteria' (same root as the female organ 'uterus') when working with women who had been sexually abused, has been instrumental in reinforcing the conclusions that women have a great deal more shame than men; in his essay Femininity he even wrote about shame as 'a feminine characteristic par excellence'.

It is a difficult question, because women and men do not talk about their emotions in the same way. Women speak more explicitly of shame. Furthermore, certain emotional states are more acceptable among women than among men, and vice versa. For example it is acceptable for a man to be angry, but not to be sad or depressed. It is acceptable for a man to feel contempt but not fear. Because the expression of emotions is gender related it is finally better to avoid endless and sterile discussions.

* * *

Culturally controlled genital sexuality

It is artificial to dissociate the different facets of orgasmophobia. However, in order to interpret its universality, we'll first focus on genital sexuality, because the organization of mating and the control of genital sexuality have been widely studied by cultural anthropologists, while the basic questions regarding childbirth and lactation have not yet been raised.

The organization of mating has easy-to-explain evolutionary advantages. We use the word 'evolutionary' in terms of survival of cultural milieus and human groups. Whatever the details of the practices controlling the relationship between the sexes and the selection of marital partners, the effect is always to reinforce the cohesion of a given human group by neutralizing or at least moderating one of the main reasons for aggressiveness among its members, that is sexual competition. Whatever the established rules, falling in love is more often than not at the limits of what is morally and culturally acceptable, since this transitory physiological folly cannot obey strict rules established by cultural milieus; it is usually considered pathological. It is obvious that all matrimonial rules interfere with the frequency and the quality of ecstatic states related to genital sexuality.

Many theories have been suggested to interpret the evolutionary advantages of particular forms of marital arrangements.[1] For example the widespread custom of marrying outside a specified group of people a person belongs to ('exogamy') has inspired the 'Alliance Theory'. In the case of exogamy, according to Claude Levi-Strauss, when small groups must force their members to marry outside the group, it is a way to build alliances with other specified groups. According to this theory groups that engage in exogamy would flourish by establishing ties for cultural and economical exchange.[2] The exchange of men and/or women therefore serves as a uniting force between specified groups. Furthermore it has also been underlined that exogamy is a way to prevent the negative effects of consanguinity.[3]

One must also theorize about the evolutionary advantages of marrying within a social group. In some cultures 'endogamy' is practiced very strictly as an inherent part of the moral values, traditions or religious beliefs. An extreme example of endogamy is found in arab countries such as Saudi Arabia, Syria, Jordan, Oman, and also Tunisia, where the number of marriages between first cousins – preferably cousins via the fathers – is high.[4] The advantages are mostly economical. It is an obvious way to maintain strong links within family clans. In general endogamy encourages group affiliation and bonding. It is a common practice among displanted cultures attempting to make roots in new countries as it encourages group solidarity and ensures greater control over group resources. It helps minorities to survive over a long time in societies with other practices and beliefs. Famous examples of strictly endogamous groups are the Yazidi in Northern Iraq (under Islamic majority), Orthodox Jews, Old Order Amish, and the Parsi, a non-Hindu minority in India

Culturally controlled childbirth

What are the evolutionary advantages of routinely adding to the difficulties of human birth?

What are the advantages of claiming that the colostrum

is bad? Of prohibiting the contact between mother and newborn baby as long as the permission has not been given by the shaman, the godfather, the father, or simply the midwife, for example? Of banning in particular the early eye-to eye contact between mother and newborn baby? Of delaying the initiation of lactation?

While volumes have been written about the advantages of the control and organization of mating, we enter an unexplored territory where childbirth and the initiation of breastfeeding are concerned. The main pioneer in this field is once more Niles Newton, associated with Margaret Mead – the first famous female anthropologist. As early as 1967, these two women raised questions about the intriguing universal beliefs about the 'bad colostrum'.[5] They suggested that depriving the newborn baby of the early colostrum might be a way to reinforce the laws of natural selection, assuming that weak babies would have difficulties to survive such habits. Today we are in a position to understand that the beliefs about colostrum are just one way among many others to ritually deviate from the physiological reference in the perinatal period. In the scientific context of the twenty-first century we have to enlarge the questions and also to suggest answers in terms of survival of civilizations.

Since the turning point of the 1970s we can refer to physiological concepts regarding the connections between birth physiology and lactation physiology. We have learnt that the human baby has been programmed to find the breast during the hour following birth.[6, 7, 8] We have accumulated data about the value of the colostrum. We have learnt that a safe delivery of the placenta, without any blood loss, implies the release of a high peak of oxytocin just after the birth of the baby, and that the release of this 'shy hormone' is highly dependent on environmental factors. We have understood that giving birth, among all mammals, implies the release of a cocktail of love hormones.[9] Multiple scientific disciplines suggest the importance of the period surrounding birth in the development of the capacity to love. In such a context we are prompted to enter unchartered territories and raise questions about the advantages of routinely disturbing the birth process, particularly of forbidding the interaction between mother and newborn baby. If such beliefs and rituals are so widespread it means that they have evolutionary advantages in spite of their enormous cost in terms of hemorrhage, maternal death, and death in infancy.

In order to suggest answers to these new and fundamental questions we must first recall that all societies one can study share the same basic strategies for survival. These strategies include the domination of nature and the tendency to dominate – even to eliminate – other human groups. It is therefore easy to accept that successful societies are those that develop to a high degree the human potential for aggression. When the domination of nature and the domination of other human groups is a strategy for survival, it is an advantage to develop the capacity to destroy life. It is an advantage to moderate the development of several facets of love, including the respect for Mother Earth. It is therefore an advantage to transmit from generation to generation beliefs and rituals, the effects of which are to interfere in a critical period for the development of the capacity to love.

These considerations are vital at the dawn of the third millennium. We are suddenly realizing that there are limits to the domination of nature. We understand the need to create a unity of the planetary village. At this turning point in the history of mankind, humanity must invent radically new strategies for survival. In order to invent such new strategies for survival we need more than ever the energies of love. This is why all the beliefs and rituals that have disturbed the physiological processes for thousands of years are suddenly losing their evolutionary advantages. This is why we have new reasons to try to re-discover the basic needs of laboring women and newborn babies.

We must be aware of the enormous difficulties we have to face in order to rediscover such basic needs. Thousands of years of culture cannot be erased overnight. It will take a long time to get rid of the aftermaths of deep-rooted beliefs and rituals. We constantly find new excuses to interfere with the physiological processes in the perinatal period. It can be via theories: for example it has been theorized that, immediately after birth, it would be beneficial to induce a 'bonding' between father and newborn baby that would be symmetrical to the mother-baby bonding, a renewed way to distract the mother during this critical period. It can be via medical requirements: for example, in many hospitals today, the cord must be cut right away and the mother cannot hold her baby in her arms without receiving the permission given by the pediatrician, as the modern agent of the cultural milieu.

We must also be aware of the fast development of physiology. If we accept to learn lessons from the physiological perspective, we'll be able, in spite of the difficulties, to rediscover and to satisfy the basic needs of laboring women and newborn babies, and to make the fetus ejection reflex more common. This will be a crucial step in the history of our species.

Culturally controlled access to transcendence

The orgasmophobic phase of the history of mankind is more easily interpreted if considered in the framework of a universally controlled access to transcendence. It is the role of religious institutions to channel the human capacity for transcendence. While they tend to neutralize physiological transcendent emotions related to the different episodes of our sexual life, religious institutions favor other routes that can be more easily organized and regulated. For example it is comparatively easy to regulate prayer. This is what all religions do, particularly the prophetic ones. Male Jews must recite the Schema twice a day, while the Islamic Salat is performed five times a day, the supplicant turning towards Mecca in a strictly specified posture, and Christian churches offer pieces of furniture (the 'prie-Dieu') that impose a particular posture for praying and that are used according to a pre-established timing. Fasting is easy to regulate. It is also possible to ritualize the use of religious music, songs, dances, and even states of trance. Many religions have included and still include in their ceremonies the use of traditional psychedelic drugs.

After reviewing many routes to transcendence and contrasting the culturally acceptable ones and those that are culturally neutralized, we are in a position to phrase a fundamental and unavoidable question: what are the evolutionary advantages of channeling access to transcendence via established religions? As usual the answer is suggested by the way we formulate the question. It seems obvious that any organized system of faith and worship tends to reinforce the cohesion of a human group. It is noticeable that – although of disputable origin – the word 'religion' is suggestive of cohesion.

Studying possible routes to transcendence finally leads us to constantly refer to the factors that make human groups 'successful'. Cohesion is one of them. Another one is the development of a certain form of aggressiveness since, for thousands of years, history has been to a great extent related to harsh conflicts between human groups. Let us dream of a time when history will be mostly about the symbiotic relationship between Humanity and Mother Earth.

11

LEGENDARY ORGASMS

Miraculous conceptions are common among legendary people, particularly when their name is associated with love.

According to legend, Aphrodite, the Goddess of Love, was miraculously conceived when Cronus severed the testicles of his father Uranus and threw them into the sea. The conception of Buddha was also miraculous and unreal: after twenty years of sterility, Maya – his mother – had a strange dream in which she saw a white elephant entering her womb through the right side of her chest, and so she became pregnant. In our cultural milieu, everybody has also heard about the pre-marital miraculous conception of Jesus involving the Holy Spirit and announced by the Angel Gabriel. It was as miraculous as the conception of John the Baptist by Elizabeth the Barren after a visitation from the Angel Gabriel. There are also numerous supernatural conceptions in Greek mythology: Asklepios, who was destined to express his compassion by finding remedies for all diseases and become the God of Medicine, was conceived when his mother was miraculously impregnated by the God Apollo. As early as the seventeenth century BC, an Egyptian tale engraved on the wall of a temple tells of the wondrous conception of a Queen. Amon, the Magnificent God, took on the appearance of the King (who had not yet been through puberty) and the heiress of the throne was conceived while the Queen was in an ecstatic state. There were also similar legends in ancient China – Pri Han, a supernatural being, appeared in human form and gave a luminous object to the wife of a king – and a son was conceived. Clearly, legendary and divine people were conceived miraculously in a great diversity of cultures.

The fact that miraculous conceptions are the rule, rather than the exception, among legendary people whose names symbolize love, and among people who are considered divine, suggests that we should interpret the word 'miraculous' and determine what the functions of miracles might be. It is easy to explain that miracles are actions and events that transcend the ordinary course of nature. Since they therefore attract attention we might conclude that this could be their first role. It is noticeable in particular that the word 'miracle' is never used in the New Testament – instead, miracles are called 'signs'. In other words, miracles are like signposts that indicate where important messages may be found in the narrative. It is as if the function of a miracle passed down over the millennia through a legend is to say: 'Look here. Open your eyes. There is a message here.'

If we consider ecstatic states routes to transcendence, the message would clearly be that all these legendary people were conceived in an out-of-space-and-time reality… in other words, in orgasmic circumstances.

Recognizing that the cultural control of childbirth has made the orgasmic states associated with the fetus ejection reflex exceptionally rare, it is also interesting to note how miraculously conceived legendary people were born, particularly those whose name is associated with love. The similarities are striking. All of them were born outside the human community, protected against the beliefs, rituals, and rules established by cultural milieus. Asklepios, the God of Medicine, was born on a mountain and found by a shepherd between a goat and a dog, surrounded by a dazzling light. Aphrodite, the Goddess of Love, was born from the foam of the waves. Buddha was born in the Lumbini Garden while his mother Maya had a rest among Ashoka blossoms. 'In delight she reached her right arm out to pluck a branch and so Buddha was born... and Heaven and Earth rejoiced', which is an explicit report of an orgasmic birth outside the human community. And of course everybody knows about the legendary birth of Jesus, which took place in a stable among mammals, also outside the human community. The legend of Jesus is a perfect case for wondering about the nature and function of a legend. When we refer to the legend of Jesus, we do not share the perspective of historians, who are in search of documents whose provenances have been authenticated. We do not share the perspective of theologians either, who are interested in systems, theories, and doctrines relating to God. Our subject is the vision of Jesus as it has been passed down over the centuries, not only by scriptures and the various churches, but also by painters, poets, musicians, and other artists, including contemporary rock-musical singers.

When we bring together all these legendary conceptions and births, we can go a step further in understanding the functions of legends. When they carry valuable messages about human nature they are more likely to disseminate and survive over millennia. Many old legends seem to have been a way for human groups to keep old messages alive through the centuries, until a time when we have all the keys to decode them. Today the study of the 'scientification of love' provides such precious keys and prompts us to re-interpret many old messages. It is as if legends take on a life of their own. Like all living organisms they are transmitted through a process of natural selection. All these legendary conceptions in an out-of-time-and-space reality and all these ecstatic births outside the human community help us to become aware of orgasmophobia as one of the most threatening aspects of an excessive domestication of human beings. They suggest questions about the future of love.

12

THE FUTURE OF LOVE:
A PESSIMISTIC SCENARIO

Thanks to many recent technical advances, love hormones have suddenly become redundant. This is an unprecedented situation that forces us to consider some alarming questions more urgently than ever.

A window

By looking at ecstatic states relating to our reproductive life we have tried to penetrate the complexity of human sexuality. Any investigation of human sexuality is in itself a window through which we can initiate an exploration of love in general. Our conclusion must be that we can see the 'scientification of orgasms' as part of the 'scientification of love'. One of the effects of these vital aspects of the scientific revolution is to raise basic but paradoxically new questions, such as: 'How does the capacity to love develop?' For thousands of years it has been commonplace to promote love, to repeat that love is important and to describe different facets of love. It is only now, since we have data at our disposal provided by scientists as different as ethologists, epidemiologists, and physiologists, that we think of phrasing new fundamental questions. All the disciplines that participate in the 'scientification of love' are converging to indicate the criticality of the period surrounding birth.

Two sorts of births

In the current scientific and technical climate, there are serious reasons to be pessimistic about the future of love. Until recently, although all societies have dramatically interfered with physiological processes over the perinatal period, women have been obliged to rely on the release of cocktails of love hormones to have babies. This is not the case today.

As far as the future of love is concerned, it is no longer essential to contrast births by the vaginal route and births by cesarean section. It is more appropriate and productive to offer a new simplified classification of births of both babies and placentas. On the one hand, there are births that involve the release of love hormones. On the other, there are births that do not involve the release of love hormones. In the latter group we must include cesareans as well as deliveries of babies and placentas controlled by the use of pharmacological substitutes for the natural hormones. The most commonly used pharmacological substitutes are drips of synthetic oxytocin which replace the release of natural oxytocin, epidurals which act as a substitute for the release of natural morphine and injections of drugs for the delivery of the placenta which replace the high peak of oxytocin women have been programmed to release immediately after the birth of the baby. Of course this is just a simplified and convenient classification. One might introduce a third intermediate group so as to include women who have a cesarean late in labor and those who receive pharmacological substitutes late on in labor. In such cases there has been the beginning of a hormonal flow, but finally the peak of the love hormone just after the birth of the baby is inhibited.

At a time when most cesareans are carried out without general anesthesia it is customary to encourage immediate skin-to-skin contact between mother and baby. The good intentions behind this policy involve trying to imitate what the first contact between mother and newborn baby might have been in the case of a non-medicated vaginal birth. However, there are inevitably enormous differences because neither mother nor the baby are in a special hormonal balance after a cesarean operation (particularly a non-labor c-section). In other words, after a birth by cesarean the hour following birth is not critical for mother-baby attachment. From a theoretical point of view, there might at least be a bacteriological advantage in immediate skin-to-skin contact because this early contact creates the conditions for an immediate colonization of the baby's body by germs carried by the mother, ie by familiar germs, since the maternal antibodies (IgG) cross the placenta. For similar reasons it might be an advantage for the baby to be in the arms of a familiar person such as the father while the mother is still on the operating table and not yet autonomous.

Such a simplified classification clearly shows that today the number of women who give birth to their babies and placentas by means of love hormones is gradually decreasing all over the world, and is even already almost negligible in many countries. The number of women who feed their babies with the help of love hormones is also reduced, since the development of formulas of 'humanized' artificial milk has made it easy for infant feeding to occur without any love hormones. Furthermore, thanks to medically assisted conception, love hormones are not even necessary to bring together sperm and egg. However, when contemplating several possible scenarios regarding the future of love we must focus on the period surrounding birth, because this constitutes the episode of human sexual life which is routinely disturbed and it appears to be a critical period in terms of developing the capacity to love.

Clearly, there are serious reasons to contemplate a pessimistic, yet highly plausible scenario. What if influential people (and consequently almost everybody) fail to notice that the redundancy of the hormones of love is an unprecedented turning point in the history of mankind? What if we ignore the most spectacular feat of the super-intelligent *Homo sapiens*, which has been to make love hormones useless? These are questions which need to be asked in as persuasive a manner as possible. Detailed prophecies are useless.

13

THE FUTURE OF LOVE:
OPTIMISTIC SCENARIOS

Reasons for hope

However, optimistic scenarios should not be dismissed. All of them are based on the hypothesis that a new awareness is possible before it is too late.

Optimistic scenarios imply that future generations will realize that the redundancy of love hormones is the most distressing aspect of the domination of Nature. After all, the most crucial questions we face are to do with our awakening to a new awareness. Everywhere in the world there are tiny cores of people – mostly women – who raise the right questions, either directly or indirectly. Conferences and seminars about pregnancy, childbirth and breastfeeding provide opportunities to meet people who are able to transcend the practical questions of daily life. They provide opportunities to meet individuals who are anxious to participate in the development of a new awareness.

However, the power of these few individuals is more

often than not limited, because many of them can only communicate what they know intuitively. They can only speak 'the language of the heart'. This is why they can only preach to the converted. In order to become really efficient they have to learn to be bilingual. This means that they must train themselves to combine 'the language of the heart' and the language of the scientific world. In particular, they must be familiar with data provided by the disciplines involved in the 'scientification of love'.

We do have cause for hope, though: the advent of a new awareness can occur in unpredictable ways at unpredictable moments. This has been the case, for example, with the new awareness which came about as a result of the epidemics of mad cow disease and foot and mouth disease. Since these epidemics were easily related to their real causes, there was a sudden new awareness of the limits of the 'industrialization of farming'.[1]

Whatever the factors are, which will eventually facilitate the emergence of a new awareness, several steps will be involved.

New criteria to evaluate the practices of obstetrics and midwifery

One of these necessary steps will be to reconsider the list of criteria needed in order to evaluate practices within the fields of obstetrics and midwifery. The short list of criteria which was established during the twentieth century has not yet been extended. This short list includes perinatal mortality and morbidity rates, maternal mortality and morbidity rates and cost effectiveness.

Until now conventional medical circles and natural childbirth movements have shared the same way of thinking. We might add the same battlefield. For example, some people within the field of obstetrics repeatedly tend to exaggerate the risks of home birth in the same way as the natural childbirth movements have a tendency to exaggerate the risks associated with cesarean sections – often emphasizing that the risk of death is multiplied by three or four after a cesarean birth, without recognizing that a cesarean is rarely the direct cause of mortality, and without taking account that the population of women who have cesareans includes a comparatively greater number of pathological conditions. Today we can overcome these difficulties. Since in most hospitals all over the world the doctrine is to perform an elective cesarean at 39 weeks in the case of breech presentations, we have at our disposal a new generation of huge homogenous statistics that make it easier to evaluate the degree of safety of the modern cesarean in well-organized departments of obstetrics. If we combine the results of a large Danish study which included 7,503 planned c-sections for breech presentation at term,[2] with a Canadian study which included 46,766 c-sections for the same reasons,[3] and the famous randomized multicentre Lancet trial (941 cases),[4] we obtain a homogenous series of 55,210 cesareans which involved not one single maternal death.

Since people within natural childbirth movements do not recognize the modern cesarean as an easy, fast and safe operation, it is difficult to go a step further. The necessary analysis of new criteria to evaluate the practices of midwifery and obstetrics is postponed. In medical circles which do not dispute the safety of the modern cesarean and which do not reconsider the conventional criteria of evaluation, the increasing rates are deemed acceptable, even welcome. This point of view has been tacitly expressed in the medical literature. For example, the author of an editorial of the *British Journal of Obstetrics and Gynaecology* has claimed that, in the near future, most women will prefer to avoid the risks associated with a birth by the vaginal route.[5] The many female obstetricians who choose to plan a cesarean for the birth of their own babies express similar points of view in a different way.[6,7] Their way of thinking will remain legitimate, or at least understandable, as long as the hot topic is not the introduction of new criteria to evaluate obstetric practices. Which additional criteria should we perhaps use?

The *quality and duration of breastfeeding* are not examined when evaluating the practices of midwifery and obstetrics. On the other hand, in the many articles about risk factors for lactation difficulties, the way in which babies are born is not usually considered. It's time we all realized that parturition and lactation are interdependent phenomena.

Until recently the fact that the maternal body prepares to secrete and release milk before the baby is born was the realm of intuitive knowledge. Today, with the language of physiologists, it is easy to explain how the hormones released by mother and baby during labor and delivery play a role in the initiation of lactation. In fact, we now have at our disposal many examples of easy-to-explain connections between birth physiology and the physiology of lactation. When we learned that the levels of endorphins increase during labor, [8,9] and that beta-endorphin is a releaser of prolactin,[10] it suddenly became easy to explain a chain of events: physiological pain is followed by a release of endorphins, which in turn is followed by a release of prolactin. Since we know that two days after birth, when the baby is at the breast, women who gave birth vaginally release oxytocin in a pulsatile way (and therefore more effective way, compared with women who have given birth by emergency cesarean section,[11]) we have another example of such connections. This connection becomes still more significant if we add that there is a correlation between the number of pulsations when oxytocin is released two days after birth and the eventual duration of exclusive breastfeeding. We can include in this new generation of studies those demonstrating that the levels of endorphins in the milk of the fourth day are much lower than expected among women who underwent a pre-labor cesarean section.[12] Clearly, one of the effects of milk opiates probably involves inducing a sort of addiction to mother's milk and the quality and duration of breastfeeding is almost certainly influenced by the amount of opiates in a mother's milk.

In spite of obvious difficulties involved in conducting randomized trials, there are several valuable clinical studies which confirm the importance of perinatal factors on the quality of breastfeeding, and still more on its duration. It has been possible in this regard to compare the effects of epidural anesthesia with or without opiates. It seemed that women who were randomly assigned a high-dose labor epidural fentanyl (a synthetic morphine-like substance) were more likely to have stopped breastfeeding six weeks postpartum than women who were randomly assigned less fentanyl or no fentanyl.[13] A Danish study compared 28 women who had a cesarean with an epidural and 28 women who had a cesarean with general anesthesia. Women who had an epidural breastfed longer (at 6 months: 71 percent versus 39 percent).[14] Almeida and Couto conducted an interesting survey about lactation among

Brazilian female health professionals whose mission is to recommend exclusive breastfeeding for six months.[15] When these experts in lactation had their own babies the average duration of exclusive breastfeeding was a mere 98 days! All these women had a guaranteed 120-day maternity leave. A 'detail' was mentioned in the report of this study: among university-level health professionals 85.7 percent had had c-sections, as compared with 66.7 percent among technical health professionals. The results of this study confirm that it is difficult to have good breastfeeding statistics in a pop-ulation of women who give birth by cesarean.

Of course, because of the huge adaptability of human beings, we must not focus on particular cases and anec-dotes. We must think in terms of statistics. I met a woman who successfully breastfed her four adoptive children! The point is that one cannot ignore the fact that the way a woman gives birth is one of the main factors influencing the length of time she is likely to breastfeed.

The way the gut flora is established as soon as the human baby is 'entering the world of microbes' has never been considered either when evaluating the practices of mid-wifery and obstetrics. Today we understand the important interactions between gut flora and immune system. We also understand that the gut flora is to a great extent established immediately after birth.

Studies within the framework of 'primal health research' are also not yet taken into account when evaluating the practices of obstetrics and midwifery. Until recently, when studying the genesis of pathological conditions or person-ality traits, genetic factors and environmental factors were usually contrasted. The general assumption seemed to be that a person's environment begins at birth. Today we cannot contrast these two groups of factors. We are learning that the expression of our genes is highly influenced by early (particularly pre- and perinatal) environmental factors. The questions are not any more about the comparative importance of the genes and of the environment. They are about the critical period for genes-environment interaction.

The Primal Health Research Database* can be used as a tool to determine the timing of such interactions. Primal Health Research is a developing branch of epidemiology which includes all studies exploring correlations between what happened during 'the primal period' and what happens later on in life. The primal period includes the period surrounding birth, as well as fetal life and the year following birth. From an overview of our database it seems clear that the perinatal period is critical in the genesis of a great diversity of pathological conditions and personality traits. In other words, we now have at our disposal a significant amount of data which suggests that the way we are born has lifelong consequences. Within the databank relevant studies can be found by selecting keywords such as 'juvenile criminality', 'suicide', 'drug addiction', 'anorexia nervosa', 'autism', 'asthma' or 'allergic disease'. Of course, all these keywords are related to issues which are of great topical interest.

We must emphasize the great scientific value of most studies included in our database. For example, in a study about the risk factors for autism, researchers considered the recorded data from the Swedish nationwide Birth Register regarding *all* Swedish children born over a period of 20 years (from 1974 until 1993). They also had access to

* www.primalhealthresearch.com

data on the 408 children (321 boys and 87 girls) who were eventually diagnosed as autistic after being discharged from hospital sometime between 1987 and 1994. Five matched controls were selected for each case and provided a control sample of 2,040 infants.[16] The risk of autism was significantly associated with events at birth, suggesting that the period of birth is critical in terms of genes/environment interaction, as far as autism is concerned. All the other studies of autism from a primal health research perspective suggest similar conclusions.

In spite of the publication of a great number of such studies, it seems that only a very small number of people, whatever their background, are ready to train themselves to think long term. This is why many of the valuable studies included in our database remain ignored, although they are about topical issues, and although they have been published in authoritative medical or scientific journals. This led me to introduce the concept of 'cul-de-sac epidemiology',[17] which refers to the type of studies we prefer to ignore. It is because of this general tendency to disregard studies which yield data which might make certain people uncomfortable, that it is difficult to include this particular 'primal health research' criterion... but it is clearly one which should be included in our list of criteria for evaluating the practice of midwifery and obstetrics.

The *specifically human cultural dimension* also needs to be taken into account when evaluating professional involvement with birth. We human beings are different from other mammals regarding the effects of interfering with the birth process. When the delivery of non-human mammals is disturbed the effects are immediately and easily detectable at an individual level. For example, when non-human mammals give birth by c-section or with an epidural, the mother is generally not interested in her babies. Among humans, on the other hand, a great deal of statistical data is needed in order to detect mere tendencies and risk factors. The reason for the increased complexity in our own species is simply that we speak and create cultural milieus for ourselves. In certain situations, particularly in the perinatal period, human behavior is less directly influenced by hormonal balances, but it is, on the other hand, directly affected by the cultural milieu. For example, a human mother knows when she is pregnant and can anticipate certain maternal behavior, while other mammals must wait until the moment when they release a flow of love hormones in order to be interested in their newborn babies.

This does not mean that we have nothing to learn from animal models. We learn which questions should be raised where human beings are concerned and we are reminded that the word 'civilization' – which suggests a specifically human dimension – should always be introduced in the question. If, for example, ewes do not take care of their babies after giving birth with epidural anesthesia, we must wonder about the future of a civilization born with epidurals, rather that focusing only on individual cases.

The need to think in terms of civilization is now perceived in some medical circles. Pr Michael Stark – the 'father' of the simplified technique of c-section – took the initiative to compile an academic book about cesareans and he asked me to write the last two chapters of this book. The title of the last chapter will be: 'What is the future of a civilization born by cesarean?' It is highly significant that the editor of this book is the pioneer who made the cesarean easier, faster, and safer than ever. Since the famous

'Einstein letter' to President Roosevelt in October 1939, the warnings about human-generated existential risks have been first expressed by those who were at the forefront of the scientific or technical advances at the root of the threat. The history of the cesarean offers a new typical example.

Reversing the current cultural conditioning

Another way to take into account the specifically human dimension is to reconsider the current negative cultural conditioning. Language is the most powerful agent of cultural conditioning. Studying our vocabulary, including the derivation of words, is therefore a necessary step to facilitating a new awareness. It is an essential step if we are to realize at which point we are brainwashed, where childbirth is concerned.

We must first recall the negative connotations, dominated by the concept of shame, associated with anatomical terms that identify the parts of the body directly involved in the birthing process. Such connotations can undoubtedly influence the way women give birth. In this respect it is important to note that language related to birth is highly disempowering. It repeatedly suggests that a laboring woman should need another person present, who is actually the active participant in the birth drama. The origin of 'obstetrics' is the Latin word 'obstetrix', which means 'midwife' and this word literally means 'a female standing in front of'. The root of terms such as 'obstetrix' or 'obstacle' is the Latin verb 'obstare' (to stand in front of). These etymological considerations suggest an ancient conditioning that a woman cannot give birth without somebody standing in front of her. Modern day-to-day language also transmits such conditioning. Most verbs related to childbirth are used in a passive form. Women 'are delivered' by a midwife or a doctor. There is no active verb in English for 'being born' (I had a problem when translating my book *Bien Naitre*: it eventually had to become *Entering the World*).

When skimming through medical textbooks or medical journals this tendency to make pregnant women and laboring women passive is obvious. Mothers-to-be are 'patients' and passive patients are usually contrasted with active care-providers. Among health professionals 'labor' is more often than not associated with 'management'. The implication is that a woman cannot give birth by herself: she needs a 'manager'. In the 20-line definition of 'midwife' provided by the International Alliance of Midwives the word 'care' appears six times, suggesting that a woman cannot give birth without a 'carer'.

There are, of course, differences in the way language is used in different cultures around the world. In Chinese the term *jie Sheng* is often used and this literally means 'delivery carried out by others'. In Russian, on the other hand, it seems that the vocabulary is less disempowering. The main verb to have a baby (*rodit*) is active and the commonly used term *rodit'sa* implies that 'I gave birth by myself'. The mothers say 'Rodila' (I gave birth) and they refer to a *rodil'ny dom*, which is a place to give birth (which has an active connotation too). Should we tentatively conclude there might be a link between the comparatively low rates of cesareans in Russia and the skyrocketing rates in Chinese cities?

In Western countries the belief in an obligatory dependency on birth attendants was reinforced during the second half of the twentieth century with the advent of schools of 'natural childbirth' directly or indirectly influenced by the Russian 'psychoprophylactic method'. As we mentioned before, this method was based on the concept of conditioned reflexes. The theoretical objective of the disciples of Pavlov was to get rid of cultural inhibitions by reconditioning women. This eventually led to the conclusion that women must learn to give birth and that they need to be continuously guided during labor.

The influence of such theories explains the emergence of 'methods' of 'natural' childbirth, as if the words 'method' and 'natural' were compatible. This is how an unprecedented and sophisticated form of culturally controlled childbirth suddenly developed. New fashionable words appeared, explicitly implying that a woman cannot give birth without the presence of a person who brings along her expertise or her energy. For example, the word 'coach' clearly indicates that the laboring woman needs the services of an expert. Those who have understood that the birth process is an involuntary process would never use the word 'coach'. In the same way, the word 'support' clearly indicates that a birth attendant must bring her energy to the birthing woman. The conditioning power of the word 'support' is enormous. Many women erroneously conclude that the more 'support' they have, the easier their birth will be. The alleged need for 'support' has been instrumental in establishing the dogma of the participation of the baby's father in the event. This widespread dogma is an eloquent symptom of a cultural lack of understanding of birth physiology.

Disempowering birth vocabulary is a feature of the whole perinatal period. Everybody has heard about 'cutting the cord', a phrase which suggests that rushing to separate the newborn baby from a passive and incompetent mother is a physiological necessity. Birth attendants follow rules and discuss the best time to 'put the baby to the breast'. Nobody knew until recently that during the hour after the birth, when the baby is in the arms of an ecstatic mother still 'on another planet' after a 'fetus ejection reflex', there is a high probability that he or she will be able to actively find the breast without help.

Moderating the powerful negative cultural conditioning appears to be an enormous task so one wonders whether it is a realistic objective. It appears still more Utopian, since it implies that we must at the same time get rid of the aftermath of beliefs and rituals that have interfered for ages with the physiological processes.

Whatever the difficulty, though, an authentic cultural revolution is certainly needed. This cultural revolution will be accomplished on the day when 'privacy' and 'protection' are the keywords in conversations, books, articles, conferences and media intervention into the birth of human babies. More generally, this cultural revolution will be accomplished on the day when it is recognized that in order to prevent the world from its self-destruction we must tackle the problem at its root. In other words, people who dream of a new renaissance must realize that the word 'naissance' is included in the word 'renaissance'.[18]

Meanwhile

Although we must expect our optimistic scenarios to become a future reality, we must also accept that thousands of years of culture cannot be erased overnight. Anyway, it is likely that, in all cultural milieus, women will always retain a level of inequality as regards personal conditioning. This is why any attempt to moderate the negative aspects of cultural conditioning must be associated with an awareness of the solution the evolutionary process has found in order to overcome the specifically human handicap. Language and cultural conditioning are related to the huge development in our species of the neocortex. In other words during the birth process (or during any sort of sexual experience) most inhibitions are related to neocortical activity. We emphasized that the solution Nature found to overcome this human vulnerability is easy to explain in the current scientific climate: during the birth process the neocortex is supposed to reduce its activity. From a practical perspective this means that a laboring woman needs to be protected from any sort of stimulation of her neocortex. This crucial aspect of birth physiology among humans was not understood by the theoreticians of the twentieth century. This is the 'original sin' at the root of the cascade of mistakes transmitted by most schools of 'natural childbirth'.

Meanwhile, women who need cesareans or drugs to have babies must not feel guilty. They must not worry about the future of their children as individuals: thanks to the cultural milieus in which they live, human beings are enormously adaptable. In fact, instead of feeling inadequate, these mothers – as well as the rest of the world! – must accept that questions should be raised in terms of civilization. All mothers, all parents, all those preoccupied by the future of humanity must participate in the emergence of a new awareness and wonder what will happen in a few generations if we continue heading in the same direction.

Today, as far as childbirth is concerned, we are like a traveler who discovers she is going the wrong way. In this kind of situation the best approach is usually to go back to where you started, before it's too late, and to try another direction. Let's hope it's not too late. Let's hope that, in spite of human ingenuity, love hormones will go on imprinting the body of our descendants. If there is a future for love, there is a future for humanity.

WEDDING-NIGHT PREPARATION

It is probable that those who do not have a scientific background could not easily understand some paragraphs of this book. However, everybody will grasp the meaning of the message sent by Sarah to her fiancé John.

Dear John,

So, in a month we'll be husband and wife. I have been introduced to Valerie, a wonderful 'wedding-night educator'. We are so advanced in our programme of wedding-night preparation that at the end of the last session I was able to write my 'wedding-night plan' (see attached file). Please read carefully the paragraph about 'positions'. I mention the positions I want you to avoid. I want you to avoid in particular position 3b. According to Valerie, this position is not natural, since it was invented by missionaries in Africa. As you know, I want to make it natural. Read also what I wrote in the paragraph 'timing'. I want the foreplays to last at least 20 minutes, but not more than 40 minutes. Valerie provides data suggesting that very fast and very long foreplays as well are not natural. I want to make it natural.

We must also choose a place for our wedding-night. As

you know, our families are pushing for a well-equipped specialised wedding-night hotel. After discussing the pros and cons with Valerie, I decided to have a home wedding-night. I hope you'll agree. I want it to be as natural as possible.

Don't forget that you are invited to participate in the next preparation session. It will be about anatomy and physiology. Valerie thinks it is essential you understand the reflex that leads to the contractions of the seminal vesicles during the sperm ejection. You must also understand how the pudendal nerves make my clitoris a highly erogenous zone, while it is thanks to the hypogastric nerves that my cervix is sensitive. We must understand how nature works if we want to make it more natural.

I am pleased that you'll have an opportunity to meet Valerie. She is such a warm, motherly, wise and erudite person. I am happy that has agreed to be close to us on our wedding-night. I'll feel more secure. She warned me against the risks of breathing too quickly during the foreplays. If she is around, she will discreetly provide her support and help me to breathe in a more natural way. I want to make it natural.

I want to make our wedding-night an unforgettable experience. I also feel the need to make a film that wedding-night educators can use in the future. This is why my old close friend Jenny will be there as well. She will come with her infrared camera, which works in the dark. In a session about physiology Valerie had explained why darkness is more natural in such circumstances. I want to make it natural.

Dear John, I look forward to hearing your comments. Let me know how you will prepare yourself for this unique event.

> I love you,
> Sarah

REFERENCES

Chapter 1
THE TOP OF THE LADDERS

1 Wilhelm Reich. *The Function of the Orgasms*. Wilhem Reich Infant Trust fund. 1942
2 Helen Deutsch. *Psychoanalysis of the sexual functions of women*. Karnac Books. London, New York 1991 (written 1923-24).
3 George Ryley Scott. *The history of prostitution*. Senate. London 1996
4 Kroll Una. A womb-centred life. In: *Sex and God*. Linda Hurcombe (ed.) Routledge and Keagan Paul, London 1987. p102
5 Niles Newton. The Influence of the Let-Down Reflex in Breast Feeding on the Mother-Child Relationship. *Marriage and Family Living* 1958; 20: 18-20
6 Pert CB, Snyder SH. Opiate receptors: demonstration in nervous tissue. *Science* (March) 1973.
7 Lederman RP, McCann DS, Work B, Huber MJ. Endogenous plasma epinephrine and norepinephrine in last-trimester pregnancy and labor. *Am J Obstet Gynecol* 1977;129:5-8
8 Michel Odent. *The Scientification of Love*. Free Association Books. London 1999.

Chapter 2
EXPLORING THE ULTIMATE STEPS OF THE BIRTH LADDER

1   Sarah Buckley. Ecstatic Birth. In: *Gentle Birth, Gentle Mothering.* One Moon Press. Brisbane 2005.
2   Newton N, Foshee D, Newton M. Experimental inhibition of labor through environmental disturbance. *Obstet Gynecol* 1966;67:371-377.
3   Newton N. The fetus ejection reflex revisited. *Birth* 1987;14(2):106-108.
4   Odent M. The fetus ejection reflex. *Birth* 1987;14(2):104-105.
5   Odent M. New reasons and new ways to study birth physiology. *Int J Gynecol Obstet.* 2001;75 Suppl 1: S39-S455
6   Odent M. Fear of death during labour. *Journal of Reproductive and Infant Psychology* 2001;9:43-47
7   Odent M. Why laboring women don't need support. *Mothering* 1996; 80: 46-51.
8   Odent M. The second stage as a disruption of the fetus ejection reflex. *Midwifery Today* Int Midwife. 2000 Autumn;(55):12
9   Lederman RP, Lederman E, Work BA, McCann DS. The relationship of maternal anxiety, plasma catecholamines, and plasma cortisol to progress in labor. *Am J Obstet Gynecol* 1978;132:495-500
10 Lederman RP, McCann DS, Work B, Huber MJ. Endogenous plasma epinephrine and norepinephrine in last-trimester pregnancy and labor. *Am J Obstet Gynecol* 1977;129:5-8
11 Wray S. Uterine contraction and physiological mechanisms of modulation. *Am J Physiol* 1993;264:C1-18.
12 Segal, Scott MD; Csavoy, Andrew N. BS; Datta, Sanjay MD. The Tocolytic Effect of Catecholamines in the Gravid Rat Uterus. *Anesthesia and Analgesia* 1998; 87(4): 864-869
13 Odent M. Birth under water. *Lancet* 1983: 1476-1477.
14 Nissen E, Lilja G, Widström AM, Uvnäs-Moberg K. Elevation of oxytocin levels early post partum in women. *Acta Obstet Gynecol Scand.* 1995 Aug;74(7):530-3
15 Lederman RP, Lederman E, Work BA, McCann DS. Anxiety and epinephrine in multiparous women in labor: relationship to

duration of labor and fetal heart rate pattern. *Am J Obstet Gynecol* 1985;153:870-7

16 Ferguson, JKW. (1941). A study of the motility of the intact uterus at term. *Surg Gynecol Obstet*. 73: 359-66.

Chapter 3
THE TURNING POINT OF THE 1970s

1 Gillett J 1979 Childbirth in Pithiviers, France. *Lancet* 2:894-896.

2 Odent M. *Birth reborn*. Pantheon. NY 1986.

3 James DeMeo. The Geography of male and female genital mutilation. In: *Sexual mutilations*. George C Denniston and Marilyn Milos ed: 1-15 Plenum Press. New York 1997

4 Schiefenhovel W 1978 *Childbirth among the Eipos*, New Guinea. Film presented at the Congress of Ethnomedicine. Gottingen. Germany

5 Eaton SB, Shostak M, Konner M 1988 *The paleolithic prescription.* Harper and Row, New York.

6 Lozoff B. Birth in non-industrial societies. In: *Birth, interaction and attachment*. Marshall Klaus, Martha Oschrin Robertson, ed. Johnson & Johnson 1982: 1-6.

7 George J. Engelmann. *Labor Among Primitive Peoples*. J.H. Chambers & Co. St. Louis 1884

8 Odent M. Colostrum and civilization. In: Odent M. *The Nature of Birth and Breastfeeding*. Bergin & Garvey 1992. 2nd ed 2003 (Birth and Breastfeeding. Clairview).

9 Odent M. Neonatal tetanus. *Lancet* 2008; 371:385-386

10 Sobonfu Somé 1999. *Welcoming Spirit Home: Ancient African Teachings to celebrate children and community*. Novato, CA: New world library

11 Margaret Mead. *Sex and temperament in three primitive societies*. William Morrow 1935.

12 Odent M. The early expression of the rooting reflex. *Proceedings of the 5th International Congress of Psychosomatic Obstetrics and Gynaecology, Rome 1977*. London: Academic Press, 1977: 1117-19.

13 Odent M. L'expression précoce du réflexe de fouissement. In:

Les cahiers du nouveau-né 1978; 1-2: 169-185

14 Michel Odent. La première têtée. In: *Genèse de l'homme écologique*. P 103-116. Epi. Paris 1979

Chapter 4
MEN ALSO HAVE ORGASMS

1 Komisaruk BR, Larsson K. Suppression of a spinal and a cranial nerve reflex by vaginal or rectal probing in rats. *Brain Research* 1971;35:231-235.

2 Komisaruk BR, Beyer-Flores C, Whipple B. *The science of orgasm*. The Johns Hopkins University Press. Baltimore 2006.

3 Higushi VS, Uchide K, Honda K, Negoro H. Pelvic neurotomy abolishes the fetus-expulsion reflex an induces dystocia in the rat. *Experimental Neurology* 1987;96:443-455.

4 Rowe DW, Erskine MS. C-fos proto-oncogene activity induced by mating in the preoptic area, hypothalamus and amygdale in the female rat: role of afferent input via the pelvic nerve. *Brain Research* 1993;621:25-34.

5 Pfaus JG, Damsa G, Wenkstern D, Fibiger HC. Sexual activity increases dopamine transmission in the nucleus accumbens and striatum in female rats. *Brain Research* 1995;693:21-30

6 Helen Deutsch. *Psychoanalysis of the sexual functions of women.* Karnac Books. London New York 1991 (written 1923-24).

7 Vance EB, Wagner NN. Written description of orgasm: a study of sex differences. *Archives of sexual behavior* 1976;5:87-98.

8 Singer J, Singer I. Types of female orgasm. *Journal of sex research* 1972;8:255-267.

9 Ladas AK, Whipple B, Perry JD. *The G spot and other recent discoveries about human sexuality*. New York: Holt, Rinehart and Winston 1982.

10 Carmichael MS, Humbert R, Dixen J, Palmisano G, Greenleaf W, Davidson JM. Plasma oxytocin increases in the human sexual response. *J Clin Endocrinol Metab.* 1987;64:27-31

11 Carmichael MS, Warburton VL, Dixen J, Davidson JM. Relationships among cardiovascular, muscular, and oxytocin responses during human sexual activity. *Arch Sex Behav.*

1994;23:59-77

12 Egli CE, Newton M. Transport of carbon particles in the human female reproductive tract. *Fertility and Sterility*, 1961;12: 151-55

13 Fox C, Wolff H, Baker J. Measurement of intravaginal and intrauterine pressure during human coitus by radio-telemetry. *J Reprod Fert* 1970;22:243.

14 Goodlin RC, Schmidt W, Creevy DC. Uterine tension and fetal heart rate during maternal orgasm. *Obstet and Gynecol* 1972;39(1):125-127.

15 Sharaf H., Foda H.D., Said S.I., Bodansky M. Oxytocin and related peptides elicit contractions of prostate and seminal vesicle. In: *Oxytocin in maternal, sexual and social behavior*. Pedersen C.A., et al (eds.) Annuals of the NY Acad. Sci. 1992;652:474-77

16 Pfaus JG, Gorzalka BB. Opioids and sexual behavior. *Neurosci Biobehav Rev.* 1987;11:1-34

17 Murphy MR, Checkley SA, Seckl JR, Lightman SL. Naloxone inhibits oxytocin release at orgasm in man. *J Clin Endocrinol Metab* 1990 Oct;71(4):1056-8

18 Exton MS, Krüger TH, Bursch N, Haake P, Knapp W, Schedlowski M, Hartmann U. Endocrine response to masturbation-induced orgasm in healthy men following a 3-week sexual abstinence. *World J Urol* 2001 Nov;19(5):377-82

19 Exton MS, Bindert A, Krüger T, Scheller F, Hartmann U, Schedlowski M. Cardiovascular and endocrine alterations after masturbation-induced orgasm in women. *Psychosom Med* 1999 May-Jun;61(3):280-9

20 Krüger TH, Haake P, Chereath D, Knapp W, Janssen OE, Exton MS, Schedlowski M, Hartmann U. Specificity of the neuroendocrine response to orgasm during sexual arousal in men. *J Endocrinol* 2003 Apr;177(1):57-64

21 Haake P, Schedlowski M, Exton MS, et al. Acute neuroendocrine response to sexual stimulation in sexual offenders. *Can J Psychiatry* 2003 May;48(4):265-71.

22 Komisaruk BR, Whipple B. Evidence that vaginal self-stimulation in women suppresses experimentally-induced finger pain. *Society for Neuroscience Abstracts* 1984;10:675.

23 Whipple B, Komisurak BR. Elevation of pain threshold by vaginal stimulation in women. *Pain* 1985;21:357-367.
24 Whipple B, Komisurak BR. Analgesia produced in women by genital self-stimulation. *Journal of Sex Research* 1988;24:130-140.
25 Evans RW, Couch JR. Orgasm and migraine. *Headache* 2001;41:512-514.
26 Levin RJ. The mechanisms of human female sexual arousal. *Annu Rev Sex Res.* 1992;3:1-48.
27 Creed KE, Carati CJ, Keogh EJ. The physiology of penile erection. *Oxf Rev Reprod Biol.* 1991;13:73-95.
28 Kimchi T, Xu J, Dulac C. A functional circuit underlying male sexual behaviour in the female mouse brain. *Nature* 2007 Aug 5; (Epub ahead of print)
29 Grammer K, Julte A. Battle of odours: significance of pheromones for human reproduction (article in German). Gynakol. Geburtshilfliche Rundsch 1997;37(3):150-3.
30 Cutler WB, Friedmann E, McCoy NL. Pheromonal influences on sociosexual behaviour in men. *Arch. Sex. Behav.* 1998; 27(1): 1-13.
31 Tiihonen, J, Kuikka J, Kupila J, et al. Increase in cerebral blood flow of right prefrontal cortex in man during orgasm. *Neuroscience Letters* 1994;170: 241-243.
32 Miller BL, Cummings JL, McIntyre H, et al. Hypersexuality or altered sexual preference following brain injury. *Journal of Neurology, Neurosurgery, and Psychiatry* 1986;49:867-873.
33 Holstege G, Georgiadis JG, Paans AMJ, et al. Brain Activation during Human Male Ejaculation. *The Journal of Neuroscience*, October 8, 2003, 23(27):9185-9193
34 Mould DE. Neuromuscular aspects of women's orgasm. *Journal of Sex Research* 1980;16:193-201.
35 Georgiadis JR, Kortekaas R, Kuipers R, et al. Regional cerebral blood flow changes associated with clitorally induced orgasm in healthy women. *Eur J Neurosci.* 2006 Dec;24(11):3305-16

Chapter 5
FROM GILGAMESH TO 21ST CENTURY AWARENESS

1   Sandars NK, translator. *The Epic of Gilgamesh*. Penguin Epics

2006.

2 Ashley Thirleby. *Tantra; the Key to Sexual Power and Pleasure*. Jaico. Bombay, 1982.

3 Jenny Wade. *Transcendent Sex: when lovemaking opens the veil*. Paraview Pocket Books 2004.

4 James DeMeo. *Saharasia*. Orgone Biophysical Research Lab. Greensprings, Oregon 1998

5 Sheila Kitzinger. *Woman's experience of sex*. Penguin 1983

6 James DeMeo. The Geography of male and female genital mutilation. In: *Sexual mutilations*. George C Denniston and Marilyn Milos ed: 1-15 Plenum Press. New York 1997

7 Fisher HE, Aron A, Brown LL. Romantic love: a mammalian brain system for mate choice. *Philos Trans R Soc Lond B Biol Sci* 2006; 361 (1476): 2173-6

8 Barlels A, Zeki S. The neural basis of romantic love. *Neureport* 2000; 11(17): 3829-34

9 Leibowitz MR. *The chemistry of love*. Little Brown, Boston 1983

10 Marazziti D, Akiskal HS, Rossi A, Cassano GB. Alteration of the serotonin transporter in romantic love. *Psychol Med* 1999;29(3):741-5

11 Marazziti D, Canale D. Hormonal changes when falling in love. *Psychoneuroendocrilogy* 2004; 29(7): 931-6.

12 Emanuele E, Politi P, Bianchi M, et al. Raised plasma nerve growth factor levels associated with early-stage romantic love. *Psychoneuroendocrilogy* 2006; 31(3): 295-6

13 Kim J, Hatfield E. Love types and subjective well-being: A cross-cultural study. *Social behavior and personality*. 2004; 32 (2): 173-182

14 Madeleine Odent. Joie. In: *Rayons du Soir*. Les Presses de Monteil. Pessac 1978

Chapter 6
THE MILKY WAY

1 Sheila Kitzinger. *Woman's experience of sex*. Penguin 1983.

2 Helen Deutsch. *Psychoanalysis of the sexual functions of women*. Karnac Books. London New York 1991 (written 1923-

24).

3   Masters, WH; Johnson, VE. *Human Sexual Response*. Toronto; New York: Bantam Books 1966

4   Donker JD, Koshi JH, Petersen WE. The effect of exogenous oxytocin in blocking the normal relationship between endogenous oxytocic substance and the milk ejection phenomenon. *Science* 1954;119:67.

5   McNeilly AS, Robinson IC, Houston MJ, Howie PW Release of oxytocin and prolactin in response to suckling. *Br Med J* (Clin Res Ed).1983 Jan 22;286(6361):257-9.

6   Nissen E, Uvnäs-Moberg K, Svensson K, Stock S, Widstrom AM, Winberg J. Different patterns of oxytocin, prolactin but not cortisol release during breastfeeding in women delivered by caesarean section or by the vaginal route. *Early Human Development* 1996; 45: 103-18.

7   Arbogast LA, Voogt JL Endogenous opioid peptides contribute to suckling-induced prolactin release by suppressing tyrosine hydroxylase activity and messenger ribonucleic acid levels in tuberoinfundibular dopaminergic neurons. *Endocrinology* 1998 Jun;139(6):2857-62.

8   Franceschini R, Venturini PL, Cataldi A, Barreca T, Ragni N, Rolandi E Plasma beta-endorphin concentrations during suckling in lactating women. *Br J Obstet Gynaecol* 1989 Jun;96(6):711-3.

9   Jones J. The mysteries of opium revealed. Oxford. Oxford University Press 1700:265. Extract mentioned by: Hawkes Ch. Endorphins: the basis of pleasure. *Journal of Neurology, Neurosurgery & Psychiatry* 1992; 55:247-250.

10 Zanardo V, Nicolussi S, Giacomin C, Faggian D, Favaro F, Plebani M. Labor pain effects on colostral milk beta endorphin concentrations of lactating mothers. *Biology of the neonate* 2001; 79 (2): 79-86.

11 Zanardo V, Nicolussi S, Carlo G, et al. Beta endorphin concentrations in human milk. *J Pediatr Gastroenterol Nutr* 2001 Aug; 33(2):160-4.

12 Dencker SJ, Johansson G, Milsom I Quantification of naturally occurring benzodiazepine-like substances in human breast milk. *Psychopharmacology* (Berl). 1992;107(1):69-72.

13 Dencker SJ, Johansson G Benzodiazepine-like substances in mother's milk. *Lancet*.1990 Feb 17;335(8686):413.

14 Odent M. Colostrum and civilization. In: Odent M. *The Nature of Birth and Breastfeeding*. Bergin & Garvey 1992. 2nd ed 2003 (Birth and Breastfeeding. Clairview).

15 Fildes VA. *Breasts, bottles and babies. A history of infant feeding*. Edinburgh University Press, 1986.

16 Rousseau J-J. *Les Confessions*. Larousse Paris 1998.

17 Kirsten Hastrup. A question of reason: breast-feeding patterns in seventeenth- and eighteenth-century Iceland. In: *The anthropology of breast-feeding*. p91-108. Vanessa Maher edit. Berg. Oxford 1992.

18 Personal correspondence with Dr Guojon Guonason. May 1993.

19 Odent M. Is promoting breastfeeding as useless as the promotion of love? *Primal Health Research Newsletter* 2003;11(1).

Chapter 7
THE UNEQUALLY EQUIPPED SEXES

1 Carmichael MS, Humbert R, Dixen J, Palmisano G, Greenleaf W, Davidson JM. Plasma oxytocin increases in the human sexual response. *J Clin Endocrinol Metab.* 1987;64:27-31

2 Carmichael MS, Warburton VL, Dixen J, Davidson JM. Relationships among cardiovascular, muscular, and oxytocin responses during human sexual activity. *Arch Sex Behav.* 1994;23:59-77

3 Jonathan Margolis. *O: The Intimate History of the Orgasm.* Arrow Books 2004

4 Terkel J, Rosenblatt, J.S. Maternal behavior induced by maternal blood plasma injected into virgin rats. *J. Comp. Physio.* Psychol. 1968; 65: 479-82

5 Rosenblatt JS, Siegel HJ, Mayer AD. Progress in the study of maternal behavior in the rat: hormonal, nonhormonal sensory and development of aspects. In Rosenblatt J.S. et al. edit. *Advances in the study of behavior.* Academic Press. NY 1979

6 Poindron P, Le Neindre P. Hormonal and behavioural basis for establishing maternal behaviour in sheep. In Zichella L,

Panchari R, edit. *Psychoneuroendocrinology in reproduction*. Elsevier-North Holland Biomechanical Press 1979

7   Rosenblatt JS. Non hormonal basis of maternal behavior in the rat. *Science* 1967;156:1512-1514.

8   Rosenblatt JS. The development of maternal responsiveness in the rat. *Am J Orthopsychiatry* 1969;39:36-56.

9   Herrenkohl LR, Rosenberg PA. Effects of hypothalamic deafferentation late in gestation on lactation and nursing behavior in the rat. *Horm Behav* 1974;5:33-41.

10 Pedersen CS, Prange J.R. Induction of maternal behavior in virgin rats after intracerebroventricular administration of oxytocin. *Pro. Natl. Acad. Sci.* USA 1979; 76: 6661-65

11 Yamaguchi K, Akaishi T, Negoro H. Effect of estrogen treatment on plasma oxytocin and vasopressin in ovariectomized rats. *Endocrinol.* Jpn 1979; 26: 197-205

12 Nomura M, McKenna E, Korach KS, Pfaff DW, Ogawa S. Estrogen receptor-beta regulates transcript levels for oxytocin and arginine vasopressin in the hypothalamic paraventricular nucleus of male mice. *Brain Res Mol Brain Res* 2002 Dec 30;109(1-2):84-94

13 Shughrue PJ, Dellovade TL, Merchenthaler I. Estrogen modulates oxytocin gene expression in regions of the rat supraoptic and paraventricular nuclei that contain estrogen receptor-beta. *Prog Brain Res* 2002;139:15-29.

14 Alves SE, Lopez V, McEwen BS, WeilandNG, Differential colocalization of estrogen receptor Beta with oxytocin and vasopressin in the paraventricular and supraoptic nuclei of the female rat brain: An immunocytochemical study. *Proc Natl Acad Sci* USA. 1998 Mar 17;95(6):3281-6

15 Jirikowski GF, Herbert Z, Petrusz P, et al. Co-expression of vasopressin and androgen-binding protein in the rat hypothalamus. *Journal of Chemical Neuroanatomy* 2005; 29 (4): 233-237

16 Zhou L, Blaustein JD, De Vries GJ. Distribution of androgen receptor immunoreactivity in vasopressin- and oxytocin-immunoreactive neurons in the male rat brain. *Endocrinology*, Vol 134, 2622-2627

17 Kerstin Uvnäs-Moberg. *The Oxytocin factor*. Da Capo Press 2003.

Chapter 8
THE HIGHWAYS TO TRANSCENDENCE

1   Maier SF, Seligman MEP. Learned helplessness: theory and evidence. *J. Exp. Psychol. General* 1976; 105: 3-46
2   Laborit H. *L'inhibition de l'action.* Paris: Masson 1980
3   Seligman MEP, Beagley C. Learned helplessness in the rat. *J. Comp. Physiol. Psychol.* 1975; 88: 534-41
4   Trimble MR. *The soul in the brain: the cerebral basis of language, art, and belief.* Baltimore: Johns Hopkins University Press, 2007.
5   Buke RM. *Cosmic Consciousness. Dulton. New* York 1969. Part 3 pp61-82
6   Deikmann AJ. Deautomatization and the Mystic Experience. *Psychiatric*, 1966; 29: 324-38
7   Liou CH, Hsieh CW, Hsieh CH, Chen JH, Wang CH, Lee SC Studies of chinese original quiet sitting by using functional magnetic resonance imaging. *Conf Proc IEEE Eng Med Biol Soc* 2005;5:5317-9
8   Chien-Hui Liou, Chang-Wei Hsieh, Chao-Hsien Hsieh, Si-Chen Lee, Jyh-Horng Chen, & Chi-Hong Wang. Correlation between Pineal Activation and Religious Meditation. *Nature* hdl:10101/npre.2007.1328.1.

Chapter 9
BONOBOS, DOLPHINS AND HUMANS

1   Frans BM de Waal. Bonobo, Sex and Society. The behavior of a close relative challenges assumptions about male supremacy in human evolution. *Scientific American* March 1995:82-88
2   Odent M. Birth under water. *Lancet* 1993;2:1376-77.
3   Michel Odent. *Water and Sexuality.* Arkana (Penguin) 1990.
4   Marean CW, Bar-Matthews B, Bernatchez J. Early human use of marine resources and pigment in South Africa during the Middle Pleistocene. *Nature* 2007 (18 Oct);449:905-908.
5   Elaine Morgan. *The Aquatic ape.* Souvenir Press. London 1982
6   Elaine Morgan. *The scars of evolution.* Souvenir Press. London 1990.

7   Elaine Morgan. *The Descent of the child*. Souvenir Press. London 1994.

8   Odent M. The primary human disease: an evolutionary perspective. *ReVision*. Washington DC 1995;18(12):19-21

9   Odent M. Plea for a new generation of research in eclampsia. Clinical Effectiveness in *Nursing* 2006; vol9. Supplement 2: e232 – e237.

10 Crawford MA, Marsh D. *The driving force: Food in Evolution and the Future*. William Heinemann. London 1989.

11 Stephen Cunnane. *Survival of the fattest: the key to human brain evolution*. World Scientific Publishing. Singapore 2005.

Chapter 10
THE EVOLUTIONARY ADVANTAGES OF ORGASMOPHOBIA

1   Thornhill, N. 1993. *The Natural History of Inbreeding and Outbreeding: Theoretical and Empirical Perspectives*. The University of Chicago Press, Chicago

2   Claude Levi-Strauss. *La pensée sauvage*. Plon. Paris 1962.

3   Morgan, Lewis Henry (1871). Systems of consanguinity and affinity of the human family. *Smithsonian Contributions to Knowledge 41*. Smithsonian Institution.

4   Youssef Courbage, Emmanuel Todd. *Le rendez-vous des civilisations*. Le Seuil. Paris 2007.

5   Mead M, Newton N. Cultural patterning in perinatal behavior. In: *Childbearing: its social and psychological aspects*. Richardson S, et al. ed. Baltimore. Williams and Williams 1967.

6   Odent M. The early expression of the rooting reflex. *Proceedings of the 5th International Congress of Psychosomatic Obstetrics and Gynaecology*, Rome 1977. London: Academic Press, 1977: 1117-19.

7   Odent M. L'expression précoce du réflexe de fouissement. In: *Les cahiers du nouveau-né* 1978 ; 1-2 : 169-185

8   Michel Odent. La première tétée. In: *Genèse de l'homme écologique*. P 103-116. Epi. Paris 1979.

7   Michel Odent. *The Scientification of love*. Free Association Books. London 1999.

Chapter 13
THE FUTURE OF LOVE: OPTIMISTIC SCENARIOS

1   Odent M. *The Farmer and the Obstetrician*. Free Association Books. London 2003 2

2   Krebs L, Langhoff-Roos J. Elective cesarean delivery for term breech. *Obstet Gynecol* 2003; 101(4): 690-6

3   Liu S, Liston RM, Joseph KS, et al. Maternal mortality and severe morbidity associated with low-risk planned cesarean delivery versus planned vaginal delivery at term. *CMAJ* 2007; 176(4) :455-60.

4   Hannah ME, Hannah WJ, et al. Planned caesarean section versus planned vaginal birth for breech presentation at term: a randomised multicentre trial. *Lancet* 2000; 356: 1375-83.

5   Steer P. Caesarean section: an evolving procedure? *Brit J Obstet Gynecol* 1998;105: 1052-55

6   Al-Mufti R, McCarthy A, Fisk NM. Survey of obstetricians' personal preference and discretionary practice. *Eur J Obstet Gynecol Reprod Biol* 1997; 73: 1-4.

7   Gabbe SG, Holzman GB. Obstetricians' choice of delivery. *Lancet* 2001; 357: 722.

8   Csontos K, Rust M, Hollt V, et al. Elevated plasma beta-endorphin levels in pregnant women and their neonates. *Life Sci.* 1979 ; 25 : 835-44.

9   Akil H, Watson SJ, Barchas JD, Li CH. Beta-endorphin immunoreactivity in rat and human blood: Radioimmunoassay, comparative levels and physiological alterations. *Life Sci.* 1979; 24: 1659-66.

10 Rivier C, Vale W, Ling N, Brown M, Guillemin R. Stimulation in vivo of the secretion of prolactin and growth hormone by beta-endorphin. *Endocrinology* 1977; 100: 238-41.

11 Nissen E, Uvnäs-Moberg K, Svensson K, Stock S, Widstrom AM, Winberg J. Different patterns of oxytocin, prolactin but not cortisol release during breastfeeding in women delivered by caesarean section or by the vaginal route. *Early Human Development* 1996; 45: 103-18

12 Zanardo V, Nicolussi S, Giacomin C, Faggian D, Favaro F, Plebani M. Labor pain effects on colostral milk beta endorphin

concentrations of lactating mothers. *Biology of the neonate* 2001; 79 (2): 79-86

13 Beilin Y, Bodian C, Weiser J, et al. Effect of labor epidural analgesia with and without fentanyl on infant breast-feeding: a prospective, randomized, double-blind study. *Anesthesiology* 2005 Dec;103(6):1211-7

14 Lie B, Juul J. Effect of epidural vs. general anesthesia on breastfeeding. *Acta Obstet Gynecol Scand* 1988; 67: 207-9.

15 Almeida JAG. *Breastfeeding: a nature-culture hybrid*. Editora Fiocruz. Rio De Janeiro 2001.

16 Hultman CM, Sparen P, Cnattingius S. 2002. Perinatal risk factors for infantile autism. *Epidemiology* 13: 417-23

17 Odent M. Between circular and cul-de-sac epidemiology. *Lancet* 2000; 355:1371.

18 Henryk Skolimoswski. The New Renaissance – Recovering from the Present Dystopia. *Network Review: Journal of the Scientific and medical network* 2007; 95: 19-22

INDEX

also from **Pinter & Martin**

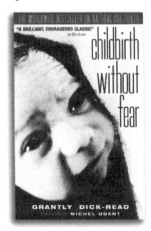

Childbirth without Fear
The Principles and Practice of Natural Childbirth

Grantly Dick-Read

with a foreword by Michel Odent

2004 | paperback | 352 pages | ISBN 978-0-9530964-6-6

In an age where birth has often been overtaken by obstetrics,
Dr Dick-Read's philosophy is still as fresh and relevant as it was
when he originally wrote this book. He unpicks every possible root
cause of western woman's fear and anxiety in pregnancy, childbirth
and breastfeeding and does so with overwhelming heart and empa-
thy. Essential reading for all parents-to-be, childbirth educators,
midwives and obstetricians!

*"When I was heavily pregnant with my first child 25 years ago this
book fell into my hands. That was the start of my belief in natural
childbirth which eventually led to four great births of my own and the
founding of my life's work in the Active Birth Movement.
Grantly Dick-Read's message is inspirational and even more relevant
today than when this book was first published. Every pregnant mother
should read it."* JANET BALASKAS – author of New Active Birth

"A brilliant, courageous classic."
INA MAY GASKIN – author of Ina May's Guide to Childbirth

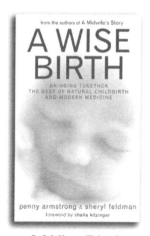

A Wise Birth

Penny Armstrong & Sheryl Feldman

2007 | paperback | ISBN 978-1-905177-03-5

What is the best way to give birth to your baby? Is it a high-tech delivery in a hospital? Or is it more naturally, at home or in a birth center? Is it possible to combine the best of modern medicine with the non-intervention of natural childbirth?

Penny Armstrong and Sheryl Feldman, authors of the wonderful *A Midwife's Story*, explore the many issues that influence the way women give birth today: culture and history, technology and psychology. They demonstrate, in a warm and convincing fashion, how to find a setting that will help make your child's birth a healthy and powerful experience.

Informative and provocative, moving and thought-provoking, *A Wise Birth* is based on Penny Armstrong's years of experience as a midwife. It is essential reading for mothers, fathers and childbirth professionals – in fact anyone interested in the politics of birth.

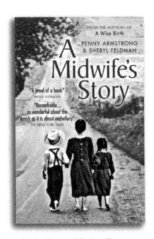

A Midwife's Story

Penny Armstrong & Sheryl Feldman

2006 | paperback | 208 pages | ISBN 978-1-905177-04-2

When hospital-trained midwife Penny Armstrong takes on a job delivering the babies of the Amish, she encounters a way of life deeply rooted in the earth. As she renews her respect for nature she discovers an approach to giving birth which would change her life for ever.

A gripping first-hand account of Armstrong's journey from student midwife in Glasgow to running her own practice in rural Pennsylvania, A Midwife's Story is a life-affirming book that never fails to enlighten, inform and surprise. Honest and ultimately very moving, it is inspirational reading not only for midwives and childbirth educators but also for all parents.

"A jewel of a book." SHEILA KITZINGER

"Remarkable ... as wonderful about the Amish as it is about midwifery." THE NEW YORK TIMES

"Penny Armstrong is a symbol of the revival of midwifery on the American continent." MICHEL ODENT – author of Birth Reborn

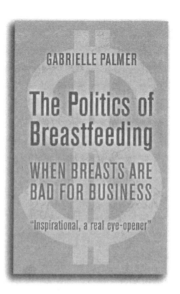

The Politics of Breastfeeding
When breasts are bad for business

Gabrielle Palmer

2009 | paperback | 400 pages | ISBN 978-1-905177-16-5

Every day more than 3,000 babies die from infections due to a lack of breastfeeding and the use of bottles, artificial milks and other risky products. In her powerful and provocative book Gabrielle Palmer describes the pressures on women, health workers and governments who are enmeshed in collusion with the sellers of infant feeding products.

An essential and inspirational eye-opener, The Politics of Breastfeeding challenges our complacency about how we feed our children and radically reappraises a subject which concerns not only mothers, but everyone: man or woman, parent or childless, old or young.

visit **www.pinterandmartin.com**
for further information, extracts and special offers